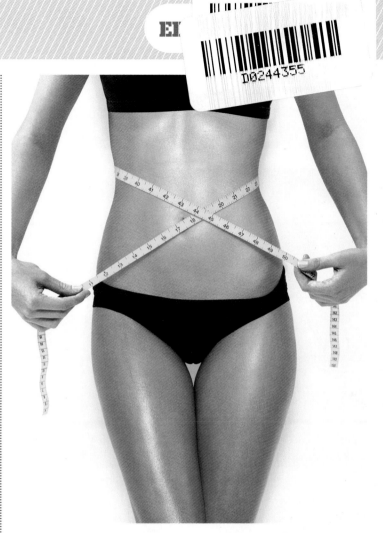

Editor
Joanna Knight
Art Director
Fanni Williams
Sub-Editors
Penny Carroll,
Ellie Moss
Contributors
Jennifer Ellis (yotopia.
co.uk), Amanda Khouv,
Ellie Moss, Louise Pyne
Pictures
Simon Taylor, Danny
Bird, Shutterstock
Cover model
Anel, motmodel.com
Workout models
Kate, Imogen, W Athletic
(wathletic.com)
**Digital Production
Manager** Nicky Baker

**Management
MagBook Publisher**
Dharmesh Mistry
Operations Director
Robin Ryan
Advertising Manager
Katie Wood
**Magbook Account
Manager**
Simone Daws
MD of Advertising
Julian Lloyd-Evans
Newstrade Director
David Barker
MD of Enterprise
Martin Belson
Chief Operating Officer
Brett Reynolds
Group Finance Director
Ian Leggett
Chief Executive
James Tye
Chairman
Felix Dennis

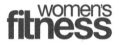

The MagBook brand is a
trademark of Dennis Publishing
Ltd. 30 Cleveland St, London
W1T 4JD. Company registered
in England. All material ©
Dennis Publishing Ltd, licensed
by Felden 2013, and may not
be reproduced in whole or
part without the consent of
the publishers.
Drop a Dress Size Bootcamp
ISBN 1781061653

**CLOTHING AND
EQUIPMENT CREDITS**
Cover: Adidas top, £28,
adidas.co.uk; Roxy bottoms,
£37, roxy-uk.co.uk
Inside: American Apparel
dress, £38, store.
americanapparel.co.uk;
Beats By Dre headphones,
£269.95, beatsbydre.com;
Green towel, Yurbuds; Gold
gloves, £99.99, and black
wraps, £3.99, both
Lonsdale, Lonsdale.com
Workouts: Reebok top,
£15, reebok.co.uk; Pineapple
bottoms, £10, pineapple.uk.
com; Asics AYAMi
ZONE, £65, asics.co.uk
Yoga workout: Pineapple top,
£12, pineapple.uk.com; Reebok
bottoms, £28, reebok.co.uk
Equipment:
physicalcompany.co.uk;
Tara Lee theyogashop.co.uk

LICENSING & SYNDICATION
To license this product,
please contact Carlotta
Serantoni on +44 (0) 20 7907
6550 or email carlotta_
serantoni@dennis.co.uk
To syndicate content from
this product, please contact
Anj Dosaj Halai on +44 (0) 20
7907 6132 or email anj_dosaj-
halai@dennis.co.uk

Dropping that elusive dress size is up there on everyone's wish list – alongside dating Ryan Gosling, swimming with dolphins and speaking several languages! But thanks to our *Drop A Dress Size Bootcamp* plan, you'll be able to tick off 'Looking hot, hot, hot in your LBD' in just four weeks. Written by our *Women's Fitness* experts, the plan is easy to follow (perfect for busy women!), and full of delicious recipes and fat-blitzing workouts.

Turn to page 7 for everything you need to get started, from fitting the plan into your schedule to finding your level. Hit our motivation station from page 19, to get in the zone and discover our secrets to acing the plan. Then, from page 30, change your eating habits for good and learn how to snack smart – you'll never look back! Armed with hot-body know-how, find your plan on page 46 and daily workouts from page 84, and get started.

Good luck... and enjoy – that elusive dress size is just around the corner!

Joanna
Joanna Knight

Contents

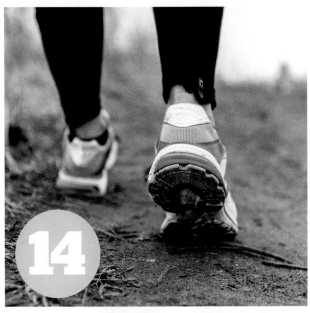

14

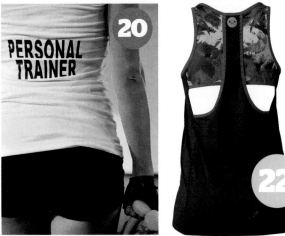

20

22

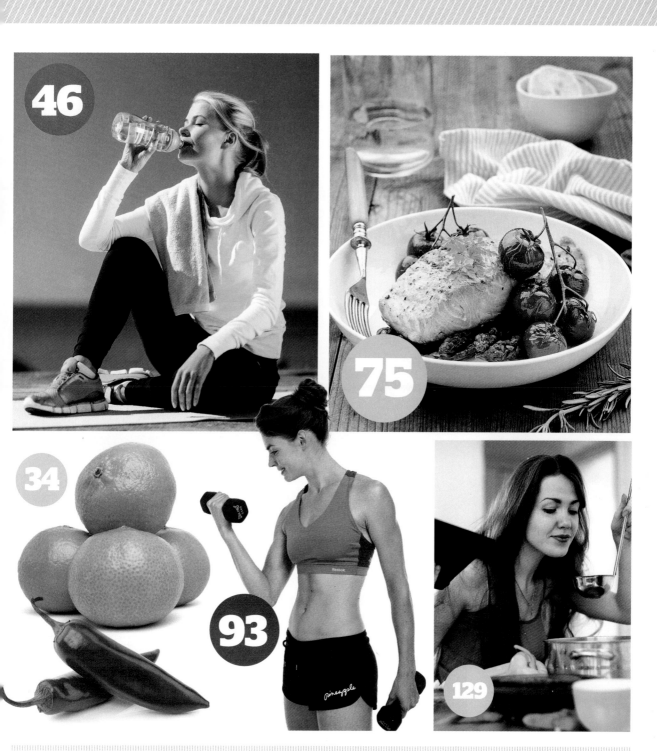

46

75

34

93

129

We are #TheEverydayActive

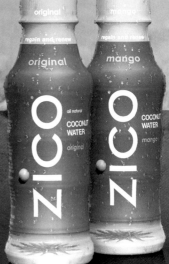

ZICO: Regain your balance. Renew your day.

ZICO is rich in potassium, the essential electrolyte that helps maintain normal muscle function, and low in calories. With zero fat and no added sugar* it's the ideal way to refresh your day. Now in a re-sealable bottle, ZICO can always be on hand so you can enjoy the benefits of coconut water throughout the day.

Find ZICO in Waitrose and selected Tesco and Sainsbury's stores and independent retailers. For more details visit zico.com/uk

*Only naturally occurring sugar from the coconuts

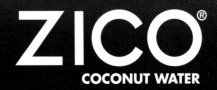

ZICO®
COCONUT WATER

 ZICOUK   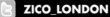 ZICO_LONDON   ZICOGB

Get started

Knowing where to start can be one of the trickiest bits of a new exercise regime. So we've put together everything you need to know to get off on the right foot

How it works

Don't do anything until you read our guide to the Drop A Dress Size Bootcamp

If you want to shift the pounds in a short space of time, you need to give it a one-two punch. The first is a healthy eating plan. The second jab is a specific training schedule. Going to the gym and just doing 'whatever' won't cut it in this case – you need a structured attack to guarantee great results. But that doesn't mean dropping a dress size can't be fun!

THE DIET

We've mapped out a healthy, achievable and – most importantly – tasty eating plan for 28 days, so you don't have to worry about what to cook, whether it's healthy enough or if it'll taste good.

The diet will provide you with loads of nutrients, giving you everything you need to balance your hormones (essential for shifting stubborn weight), boost your metabolism and balance your blood sugar to prevent fat storage. It might sound complicated but we've made sure it's easy to follow and simple to prepare. We're shattering the myth that healthy eating is boring, bland and time-consuming!

THE EXERCISE

Any exercise is better than no exercise, but when your goal is as specific as dropping a dress size in four weeks, it's time to take it up a notch. Structuring your training over the week gives you direction *and* motivation. 'Following a training plan allows you to maximise your workout in the time you have,' says Anwar Gilbert, fitness manager at The Third Space in

What to expect

Ready, steady, go girl! Enjoy these body benefits on us...

1 Furious fat burn
A mix of metabolism-boosting cardio intervals and muscle-building resistance will send your fat burn through the roof. Make the most of it by sticking to healthy food, too. You can't out-train a bad diet!

2 Mega muscle tone
The resistance plans we've devised will sculpt and tone your body, from your shoulders to your calves! As the fat melts away, you'll find a shapely new you staring back from the mirror.

3 Bundles of energy
A clean diet teamed with endorphin-enhancing exercise will work wonders for your vitality. You'll need it for all the jumping for joy you'll be doing with your new body!

'A structured plan guarantees results, but that doesn't mean it can't be fun'

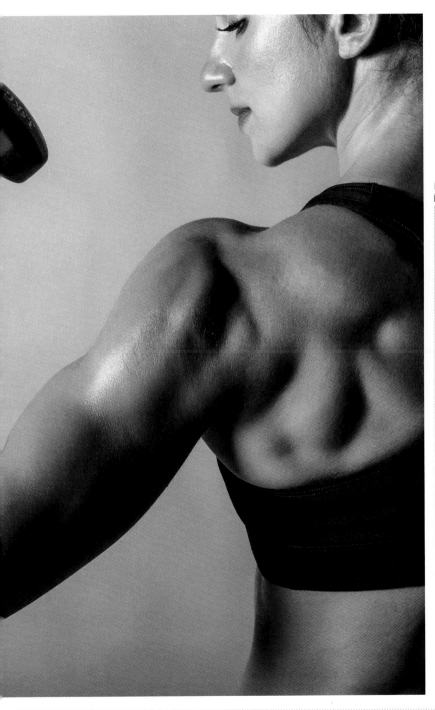

London. 'Being consistent in your training increases the chance of reaching your goals and helps keep you on the wagon.

'The odd bit of exercise here and there is great,' he continues, 'but if you have no direction in your workouts going ahead, you're less likely to hit your goals. Training on a four to six-week plan means you can change it up at the end of that phase and prevent your body hitting a plateau.'

Why a bootcamp?

Not convinced you need the full treatment to shed the kilos? Here's proof an ultimate overhaul works

'For years I've been an avid gym fan, thinking that was enough to get me my dream body. A bootcamp forced me to sync my exercise with healthy eating and rest – and, voilà, my body just started transforming.'
Tracey, 35, Berkshire

'A bootcamp is the perfect scenario if you're looking to lose weight for an event as it promotes the right kind of exercise. A structured plan encourages me not to cheat myself when I create my own routine.'
Sally, 29, York

'When I was younger, I found that I could get away with a bit of exercise now and again; eating well part of the time and whatever I fancied the rest. I re-evaluated everything after I turned 40 and found that you need to be organised in order to keep your body young.'
Anne, 46, Hertford

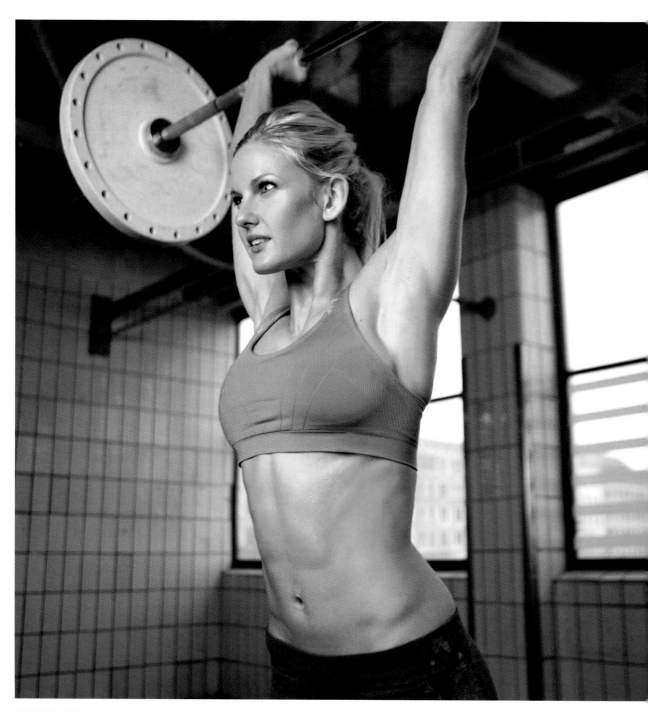

Burning questions

Want expert advice about losing weight? Personal trainer Jessica Wolny answers your FAQs

Q Why is weight training good for weight loss?

A few reasons. Firstly, getting stronger lets you move faster, shift more weight, and generally burn more calories in less time, than steady state cardio.

Secondly, weight training builds lean muscle, which needs fuel – meaning you continue to burn fat long after you leave the gym. Finally, weight training has a whole host of beneficial hormonal effects that running doesn't – it minimises cortisol, increases testosterone, and generally makes you look awesome.

Q I eat well and exercise regularly – so why am I still not losing weight?

Firstly, it's worth checking that you really *are* eating well. Try keeping a food diary for a couple of days to check that you aren't getting a huge hit of hidden sugar or calories from innocent-seeming food.

Secondly, build-up of the stress hormone cortisol can lead to fat storage – minimise it by sleeping more, and better. One good tip is to stay away from the television – and, in fact, all electronic devices – for an hour before bed, so your brain isn't buzzing with stimulation.

Q I always seem to crave sugary treats in the afternoon. Why is this?

Sugar cravings are usually a sign of tiredness – your body is looking for a quick hit of energy, and it doesn't get much quicker than chocolate or cake. Unfortunately, you'll also burn through this sort of food quickly, and the resulting insulin dump will make things even worse.

Instead, head off the sugar craving by eating low-glycaemic index foods (like

'Keep a food diary to check that you aren't getting a huge hit of hidden sugar or calories'

vegetables) at lunch, and drinking plenty of water. If you're still getting the munchies, keep a healthy snack handy: a few celery sticks with almond butter, or a handful of almonds will give you slow-release energy without derailing your fitness efforts.

Q Why does exercise make me hungry and what can I do about it?

Your body is simply trying to replace the energy it used to work out, which is perfectly normal and natural. The trick is to avoid calorie-packed foods that'll make you even hungrier – stick to a good mixture of lean protein (preferably from meat or eggs) and vegetables.

Q How much protein do I need after a workout?

Opinions differ on how much protein you can use from a single meal, but a good rule of thumb is 20-30g – it'll fill you up, prevent sugar crashes, and help you build lean, toned muscle. Most protein shakes have roughly this amount of the good stuff – as does one large chicken breast.

Q A friend of mine lost lots of weight, but when I followed the same workout routine and diet, it didn't work for me. What went wrong?

Were you really doing exactly the same thing: using similar weights, running at similar speeds, sticking to the rest periods, and resisting the urge to snack or put sugar in your daily venti latte?

If so – and if you started from a similar point – then look at other factors that may be responsible. Stress at work and poor sleep could be sabotaging your efforts.

Q Why do my muscles ache after a workout and how can I avoid the pain?

Exercise causes micro-tears in your muscle fibres. But when they repair themselves, they come back stronger.

To help the process, make sure you're fuelling up with plenty of protein and nutrients. You can also combat soreness by doing an 'active recovery' workout that flushes refreshing blood through the affected area – for instance, if you've just

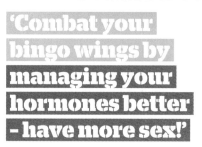

'Combat your bingo wings by managing your hormones better – have more sex!'

done a hard legs session, try a brisk walk or a very gentle jog to get that flow on.

Q Can I lose weight from a specific area of my body?

Maybe. You certainly can't 'spot-reduce' fat by exercising the affected area, but there is some evidence that you can

target weight loss by managing your hormones better. Belly fat, for instance, is linked to high cortisol levels so try yoga to chill out. While saggy arms can be from a lack of testosterone – combat these with plenty of heavy resistance exercise!

Q How much water should I drink each day when I'm exercising?

It depends how much you sweat! Assuming you're already drinking one or two litres of water a day, the best way to work this out is to weigh yourself in your workout kit before and after your workout, then make sure you're glugging the difference in water. Lost 0.5kg? Drink 500ml extra water! Easy.

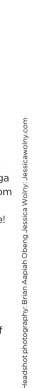

Headshot photography: Brian Aapiah Obeng Jessica Wolny: Jessicawolny.com

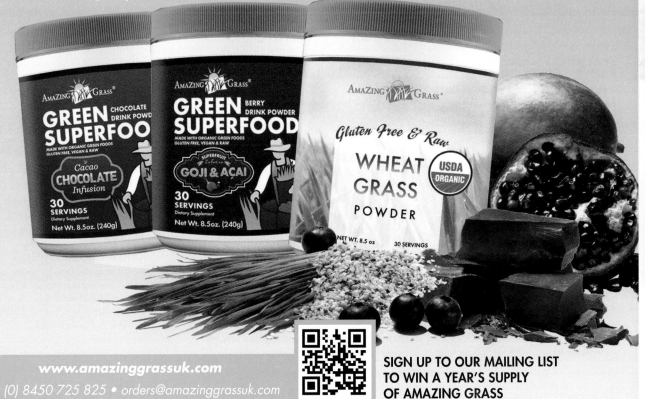

The busy girl's guide to fitting in fitness

No time? No worries! Here's how to fit this bootcamp into a jam-packed diary

Need a few more hours in the day? Who doesn't! Hectic jobs, back to back catch-ups and family demands can leave you feeling like the biggest loser when it comes to exercise. But, with a few clever tweaks, you can maximise your time to ensure you get fit and look fab, too. It's easier than you might think...

DON'T KNOW WHERE TO START? BE POSITIVE

First of all, you need to believe you can find the time to work out. Having a positive approach to your training and thinking, 'Yes, I *can* find half an hour a few times a week,' or 'I really want to squeeze in a quick workout some mornings,' is a much better way to ensure you reach your goals than saying, 'I'm just too busy.'

SEEMS TO DAUNTING? START SMALL

Make things easy for yourself and be realistic about the time you can afford to give to your workouts. Don't blithely schedule hours of workouts if you know you simply won't be able to commit to them. Start small and wedge in 30 minutes after lunch or 20 minutes in the morning. Then, when you get into the swing of things, you might find you can

squeeze in a few more sessions or make your workout a little longer. Our workout handbook – beginning on page 84 – has a super-speedy 10-minute circuit that's ideal when time starts to get a bit tight.

'Combine fitness and socialising to save those precious hours in your week'

CAN'T COMMIT? WRITE IT DOWN

It's easy to sack off sessions if you aren't fully committed to doing them. Write your workouts in your diary, tell your friends or family when you're planning to do them and tweet about upcoming sessions. It's a simple way to stay accountable.

WANT TO SEE YOUR MATES? MAKE IT SOCIAL

Why not try combining socialising and fitness to save those precious hours in your week? Invite your mates to join in your workout or meet them in the park and catch up between burpees! You could even stop off for a healthy smoothie and

a gossip afterwards. It's a great way to save time, but it'll also make it fun and help you stick to your training.

DON'T KNOW WHEN TO FIT IT IN? SIMPLES – GO EARLY!

OK, so the thought of getting up early may not sound appealing, but exercising in the morning can be a great time-saver. You'll get in a great workout, feel energised by the time you get to the office *and* you can enjoy some peace and quiet while everyone else slumbers. Plus, it leaves lunchtimes and evenings free for socialising, stretching your legs and getting fresh air – or simply chilling out!

15-minute magic!

When time is tight, try a Tabata-style session: 20 seconds of hard work, 10 seconds of rest. Try burpees, squat jumps, sprints or mountain climbers – just make sure it's a full-body move to get your heart pumping. The only rule is to work absolutely flat out in those 20 seconds. Repeat this sequence for 10-12 minutes, then hit your abs for the last few minutes. Turn to page 101 for speedy moves.

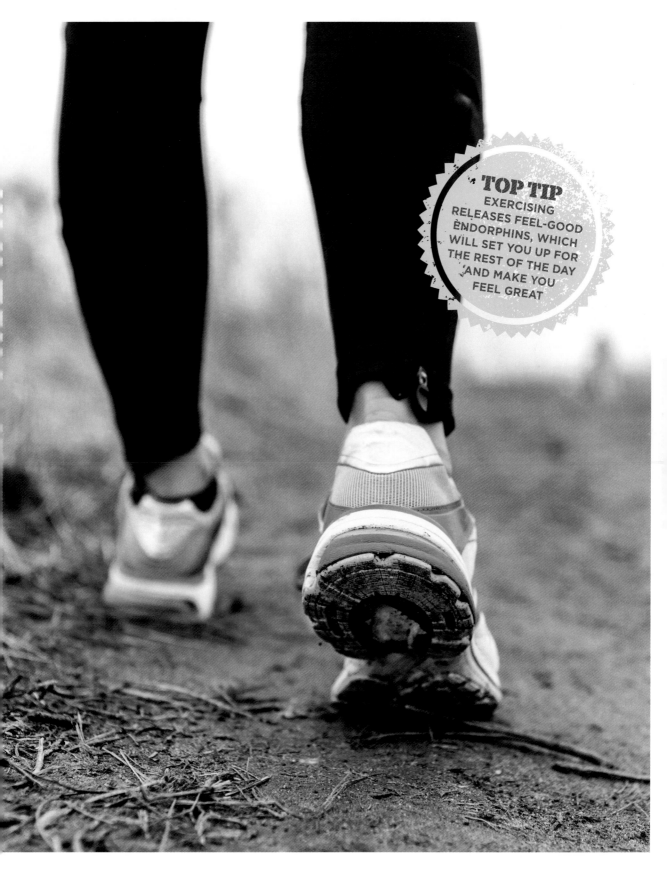

TOP TIP
EXERCISING RELEASES FEEL-GOOD ENDORPHINS, WHICH WILL SET YOU UP FOR THE REST OF THE DAY AND MAKE YOU FEEL GREAT

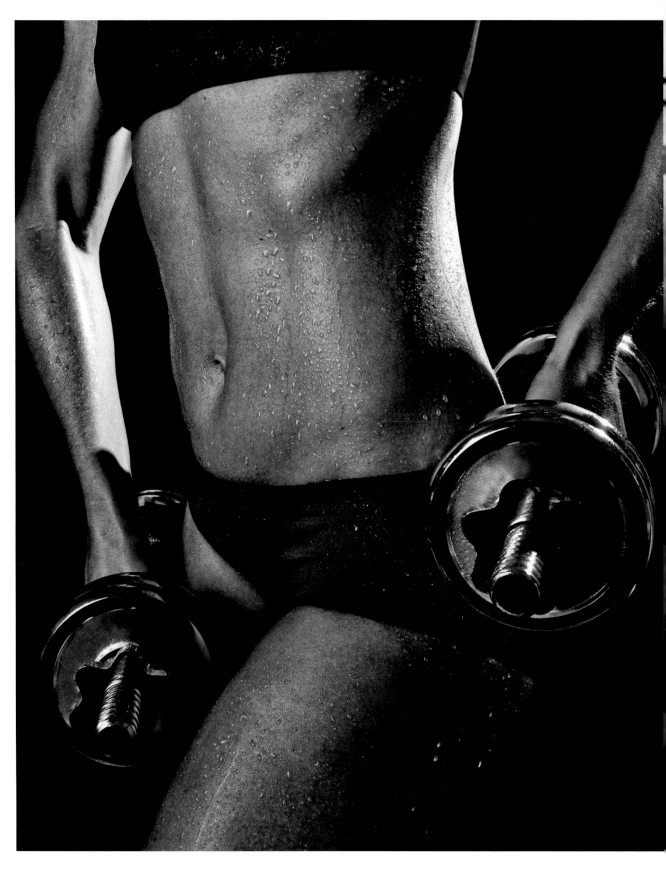

Find your level

Whether you're a fitness fresher or a seasoned gym veteran, we help you make the most of every Drop A Dress Size workout in this book

TURN TO PAGE 84 FOR YOUR WORKOUT HANDBOOK

We haven't missed a trick with this training regime. From the best type of cardio sessions to resistance workouts that rule the roost, we've got it covered. Here's what you need to know to ace all your sessions, whatever your level.

HEAVY DUTY

In this plan, we encourage you to use heavy weights, in relation to your strength, when resistance training. This weight will change depending on the move you're doing – for example, you'll be able to lift far more weight with a deadlift than, say, a shoulder press. However, you should opt for the heaviest weight you can manage for the suggested number of reps, while maintaining top-notch form.

The weights you use will, of course, vary depending on your strength, so it might take a few sets to find out which ones suit you. You should start to really feel the struggle on the last few reps of each set, but at no point should you feel in pain.

Starting light and increasing the weights will help you realise your strength as a beginner. Be sure not to go too light, though – subjecting your muscles to tension is what makes the difference.

So, push yourself, but don't take risks that could have long-term consequences. If you're not sure where to start, we've suggested weights for each workout.

FAST AND SLOW

Interval training is a no-brainer for weight loss. While steady state cardio burns calories during the workout, sprint intervals really rev up your metabolism, keeping it ticking over all day – even after you've stopped exercising.

This technique involves going as hard and fast as you can for a short period – the

'Interval training is a no-brainer – sprints rev up your metabolism'

'sprint' – followed by a slower window of recovery. You then repeat the sequence for a set time. The recovery periods are important as they allow you to put in the work during the sprint – and that's the part that really boosts the fat burn. If you can't put everything into your sprints, you won't get the same results.

You can do intervals as part of any kind of cardio training. This plan suggests you perform intervals while running or using a stationary bike, rower or cross-trainer. If you're new to it, here's what to do...

BEGINNER:

Your 15-minute cardio interval sessions should consist of 30-second sprints (as fast as you can manage for 30

seconds) followed by 60-second recovery intervals (these should be done at a slow pace, allowing your heart rate to gradually return to normal).

INTERMEDIATE:

Your 20-minute cardio sessions should consist of 30-second sprints followed by 45 to 60-second recovery intervals.

ADVANCED:

Your 20-minute cardio sessions should consist of 30-second sprints followed by 30-second recovery intervals.

All levels: make sure you warm up before you start by starting slow and gradually increasing your speed for a few minutes before you begin the intervals.

What's your level?

1 You're a beginner if...
...you've never done more than a quick run for the bus.

2 You're intermediate if...
...you regularly enjoy a range of different workouts.

3 You're advanced if...
...you've got years of training under your belt and it takes a lot to challenge you.

NEED A NATURAL LIFT?

contains fruit juice

Natural Energy Drink

delicious orange & passion fruit

refreshing cranberry & apple

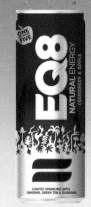

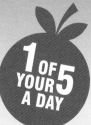

1 OF YOUR 5 A DAY

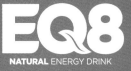

Motivation station

The key to successful weight loss is to never give up. So we've put together hot kit, a fab playlist and top tips to boost your motivation when the going gets tough

Be your own PT

Yes, you can be your own all-in-one instructor, army commander, motivation machine and nutritionist

Enlisting a personal trainer will undoubtedly see your fitness soar, but we can't all afford the luxury of weekly sessions with a superwoman or man in lycra. Fortunately, they're not exclusive purveyors of a magic weight-loss recipe. The truth is, you already have all the tools you need to smash your best body goals. Here's how to tap into your inner motivator to get real results.

SET THE SCHEDULE

Set a goal for each week and each month, and write it in your diary. This is the best way to remind yourself why you're sweating it out. Note down each session and cross it off when you're done. Looking back at all those crosses at the end of the week should make you proud!

MEASURE UP

Take your vital stats and track them each week to monitor your progress. 'Measure waist, hips, biceps, thighs, number of press-ups you can complete in a minute, number of sit-ups in a minute, how long it takes you to run 5K, your BMI, your body fat percentage and your blood pressure,' says personal trainer Mollie Millington (ptmollie.com). Check back every six to eight weeks to see how you're doing.

KEEP A FOOD DIARY

Take note of everything you eat and review it at the end of the week. Don't beat yourself up if you had a few slip-ups, but *do* note where you fell off the wagon and look for solutions to prevent the same thing occurring. If, for example, you caved in to cake in the afternoon, maybe you didn't eat enough protein at lunch.

DON'T BE A SLACKER

Analyse your performance just like a PT would. Did you have great form? Could you go heavier? Note it down and create action points for your next session. And remember you need to be working hard.
  'You can use the "rate of perceived exertion" scale or talk test to measure your intensity,' suggests Mollie. 'If you can talk in long sentences while working out, you need to pick up the intensity. If you can't speak at all, you need to ease up.'

'You already have all the tools you need to smash your body goals'

GET TECHY

Invest in a gadget like the Jawbone UP band (£99.99, jawbone.com), which works with an app to monitor your activity, food intake and sleep. This clever gadget – one of several similar ones on the market – also draws links between your behaviour patterns (a lack of sleep and overeating, for example) and sends you handy hints on how to improve.

BE YOUR OWN INSTRUCTOR

In this book we encourage you to be your own PT; setting goals, keeping food diaries, monitoring intensity and measuring up. These simple progress checks will help you see great results on this programme, plus they're key skills for keeping your fitness on track in the future.

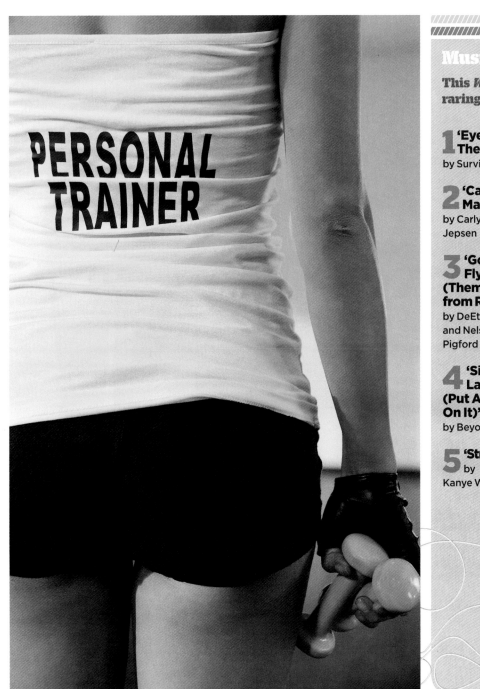

Musical motivation

This *WF* playlist will get you raring to go. Crank it up!

1 'Eye Of The Tiger' by Survivor

2 'Call Me Maybe' by Carly Rae Jepsen

3 'Gonna Fly Now (Theme from Rocky)' by DeEtta Little and Nelson Pigford

4 'Single Ladies (Put A Ring On It)' by Beyonce

5 'Stronger' by Kanye West

6 'Don't Stop Believin'' by the *Glee* cast

7 'Lose Yourself' by Eminem

8 'Seven Nation Army' by The White Stripes

9 'All The Small Things' by Blink-182

10 'We Built This City' by Starship

Go shopping!

Nothing gets your heart pumping like a brand new workout wardrobe. Try this stylish kit for size

1 BAND AID

This simple, pretty band is essential for keeping those pesky flyaways out of your eyes when you're working up a sweat – and it's non-slip too. We love! **Sweaty Betty skinny seamless headband, £8, sweatybetty.com**

2 TOP NOTCH

This layered top is the perfect way to make your workouts that little bit more special. We love the cutout, patterned back and flattering black front panel. **Roxy Outdoor Fitness Revolution top, £30, roxy.com**

3 THE RIGHT STRIPES

The stripe on these leggings is super funky – and they're so comfortable and breathable, they feel like a second skin. Win-win! **Striders Edge E-Tight, £45, stridersedge.co.uk**

4 HOT STEPPER

These lightweight and flexible training shoes offer great support, whether you're on the road or the treadmill. We love the black mesh and coral combo too! **Ecco Biom Evo Racer Ladies, £100, shopeu.ecco.com**

5 HEAR THIS

The clever design of these headphones means they 'lock' into your ears and don't fall out, no matter how intense your workout. Plus this range are designed for small ears. **Yurbuds Inspire For Women earphones, £34.99, runnersneed.com**

6 SUPPORT SYSTEM

Keep your best assets in great shape with this fab underwired, moulded sports bra. It uses Coolmax technology to wick moisture and keep you comfortable. Plus it comes in a fab shade with matching shorts, too. **Freya Active Hot Crimson sports bra, £36, freyalingerie.com**

7 STAY FRESH

Every wardrobe needs a simple, stylish vest that goes with everything. This top uses Kleanfit technology, which helps to prevent bacterial build-up, keeping you fresh all day. **HPE Classic vest, £35, hpe-shop.com**

8 SHORT SHIFT

These eye-popping shorts will add a burst of colour to your day. Team with the Roxy top for real wow factor! **Moving Comfort Momentum shorts, £31.49, prodirectrunning.com**

9 LEG IT

Up the glam factor with some fun patterned leggings. They're guaranteed to lift your mood no matter how early your workout! **Do Flash Pattern capris, £30, prodirectrunning.com**

10 BARE ALL

The barefoot training shoe gets a delicate, feminine twist. They're available in five colour combos. **Vibram FiveFingers Alitza, £79, primallifestyle.com**

Kit out your kitchen

These genius cooking tools take the fuss out of healthy eating

1 STAY CLEAN
This eco-friendly frying pan uses non-stick surface Thermolon to stop toxins leaching into your food. **GreenPan Milan 3D Frying Pan, £35, green-pan.co.uk**

2 SMOOTH OPERATOR
Create smoothies in a flash with this 600ml blender – then take them with you, as the blender chamber doubles as a bottle! **Blend Active Bottle, £29.99, breville.co.uk**

3 CUT ABOVE
Shred, slice, dice and grate in seconds with this multitasking kitchen must-have. **Tefal Fresh Express Max, £79.99, homeandcook.co.uk**

4 THE GOOD JUICE
Whizz up nut butters, purées, frozen fruit sorbets and, yes, juices with this clever machine. **Omega 8006 Juicer, £289, ukjuicers.com**

5 HOT BUY
Lock in food's natural nutrients with this nifty three-tiered steamer. Its ingenious nine-litre capacity means you can steam meat, fish, veggies and rice in one go. **Russell Hobbs 3-Tier White Food Steamer, £24.99, amazon.co.uk**

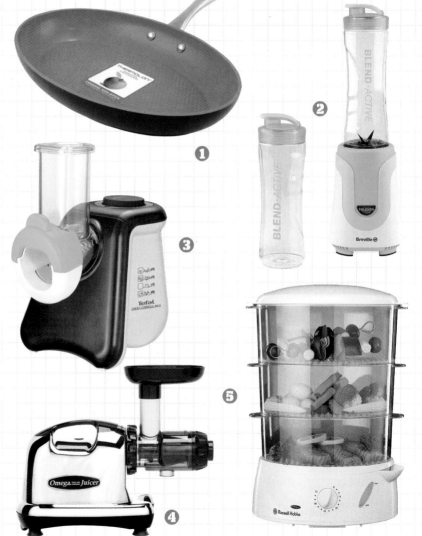

Take a break

Find out why less really is more when it comes to working out

It's one thing being dedicated to your workout schedule, but if you want to bounce back and be fighting fit for every session, you need to give your body adequate time to recover.

Research by the University of Alabama found less time in the gym could yield better results: women exercising two to four days a week burned more calories at rest than those training six times a week.

Overtraining can mess with levels of hormones such as oestrogen and cortisol, hamper your sleep, increase your risk of

'A weekly day of rest can keep you mentally focused and lift your mood'

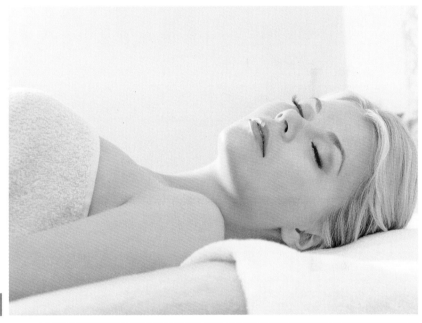

injury, and leave you feeling exhausted and vulnerable to food cravings. In contrast, a weekly day of rest can keep you mentally focused, lift your mood and help you dodge a weight-loss plateau.

A balanced diet will supply your body with the nutrients it needs to repair. Load up on anti-inflammatory foods like salmon, fruit and veg to combat damage and nosh on protein-packed eggs, chicken and pulses. And consider active recovery (working out at 50 per cent of your max effort) with a brisk walk. This helps eliminate waste products that build up in your muscles and create soreness. So the key is to take things easy!

3 ways to chill out
Use these tips to make the most of your time off

1 Get enough sleep
Aim for a seven to eight-hour slumber to feel revitalised and raring to get back into your routine. Sleep in a darkened room to improve sleep quality.

2 Help your body recuperate
Book a sports massage for the day after a hardcore workout. A well-trained practitioner will help to speed up the recovery process, easing tight muscles.

3 Soothe tired muscles
Go to the gym, but skip the weights and cardio machines and head straight to the sauna and jacuzzi for a relaxation session with muscle-boosting benefits.

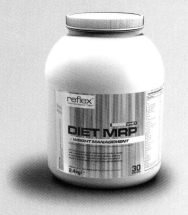

IT'S ALL IN THE
NUMBERS

44.8^g
Carbohydrate

175^{mg}
Magnesium

37.5^{mg}
Vitamin C

31^{µg}
Vitamin K2 MK-7

6.2^{µg}
Vitamin D3

7.5^{mg}
Vitamin E
(DeltaGold®)

40^g
Protein

per 100g

Eating a healthy calorie controlled and balanced diet whilst living a modern lifestyle is not always possible. Diet MRP® replaces a complete meal and provides a guaranteed balance of protein, carbohydrate and fat in conjunction with a broad spectrum of vitamins, minerals and antioxidants.

It contains low glycemic index carbohydrate sources; oats, barley and trehalose. Lower GI sources of carbohydrates are broken down slowly, providing energy over a longer period of time, allowing for a more balanced release of energy than simple carbohydrate sources such as dextrose or sucrose, which are used extensively in many cheaper meal replacements. Additionally, oats and barley are rich in other nutrients such as fibre and naturally occurring vitamins and minerals.

Diet MRP® contains a unique multivitamin and mineral complex, which is simply not found in other meal replacements. Each serving of Diet MRP® contains high quality amino acid chelated minerals; there are no cheap oxide forms of minerals like magnesium oxide or zinc oxide. You will also find the very rare form of vitamin E called DeltaGold® delta-tocotrienol and MenaquineGold™ vitamin K2 MK7. A full vitamin B complex is also present, with the addition of LactoSpore® pro-biotics.

£39.99
 www.reflex-nutrition.com

www.reflex-nutrition.com

 @ReflexNutrition

 Reflex Nutrition Ltd

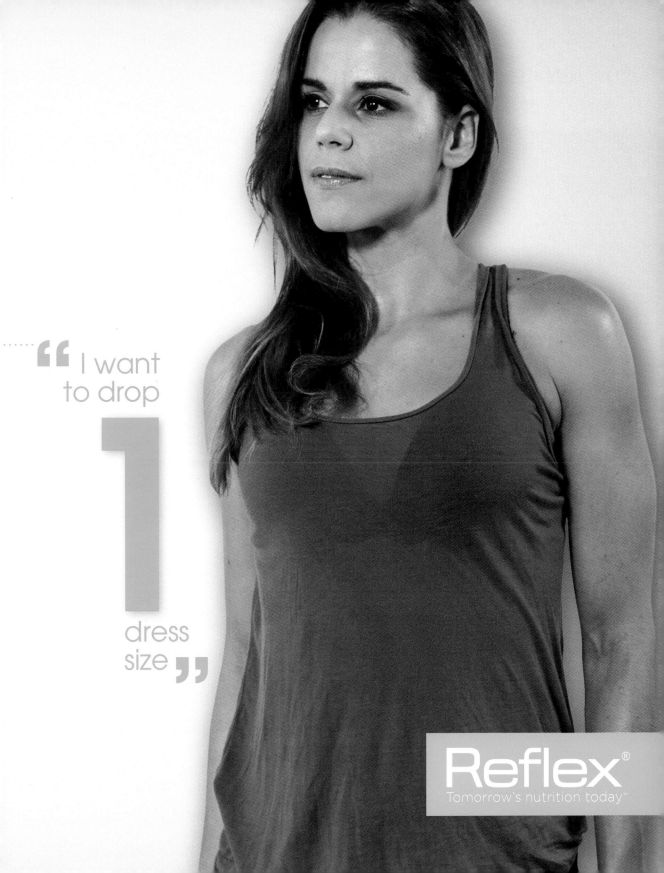

Your mouth at its best

Clinically proven range. Developed, used and recommended by dental professionals.

DEVELOPED, USED
AND RECOMMENDED
**BY DENTAL
PROFESSIONALS**

Eliminates bad breath

Stronger, whiter teeth

Gentle on teeth and gums

Fights plaque and tartar

Sulphate free

ultraDEX®
LOW-ABRASION TOOTHPASTE

FORMERLY
[retarDEX]
SAME EFFECTIVE FORMULA

ultraDEX®
LOW-ABRASION TOOTHPASTE

ultra
DEX

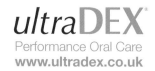

ultraDEX®
Performance Oral Care
www.ultradex.co.uk

Eat right

Great nutrition is essential for any fat-loss programme. Check out our top slimming foods, savvy swaps and cheat day tips to help you stay on track

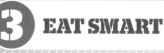

Super slim-down secrets

Find out how you can fine-tune your body to ditch the pounds for good

Smart weight loss is a no-brainer. Fad diets may offer a seemingly quick fix. But, if you want to lose weight and keep it off, you'll need to be truly savvy. If you've tried every diet under the sun and failed, it's likely that you're following the wrong rule book.

Over the next few pages, we'll uncover the real secrets to long-term, lasting weight loss – they'll help you sculpt the body you've always wanted.

A slim figure and glowing skin comes from within. Overhauling your diet and keeping active will maximise your calorie burn; nourishing your body's lymph and digestive systems, and the liver, will get your weight-loss firing on all cylinders.

It's important that these systems are functioning properly as they are your body's main channels of waste elimination. You'll learn more about this over the next few pages, but the main message is that if you want to ward off pesky spots and flaunt those enviable washboard abs, think from the inside out!

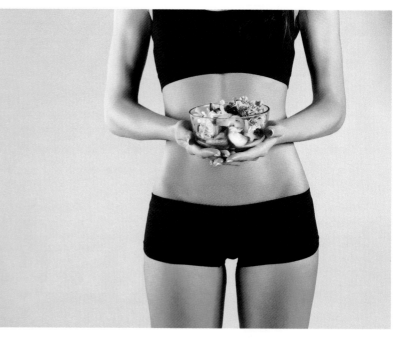

POWER OF HORMONES

There are many factors at play when it comes to weight, but hormones are probably number one. Dealing with stress for long periods can raise the hormone cortisol, which is linked to fat around the middle, and a lack of nutrients such as B and C vitamins. High cortisol can result in poor sleep and if you're not getting your eight hours every night, the appetite-stimulator ghrelin goes into overdrive.

MAINTAINING BALANCE

Controlling the hormone insulin is also crucial for effective weight loss. Insulin's job is to keep your blood sugar balanced, so you don't succumb to those pesky food cravings. So, if your insulin levels are spiralling out of control, giving in to cravings and weight gain are inevitable.

If the thought of managing all this seems a bit overwhelming, don't worry. We'll be with you every step of the way as you transform your body for good!

Treat your tummy

Get your digestion running smoothly to lose those love handles

Good health starts with good digestion and if your gut health is suffering, chances are it will show on the outside. Stubborn skin complaints, hard-to-shift pounds and a tendency to catch every bug going are key signs you need to scrutinise your body from the inside out.

The digestive process begins the moment food touches your lips. After food is swallowed, it travels down your oesophagus and into your stomach. From there it passes through the small intestine

> **'Your digestion plays a huge role... and sometimes it needs a little help'**

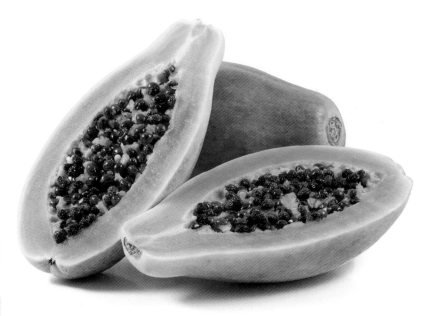

and into the colon, where it's finally expelled as waste. As food goes through each stage it's churned and broken down to keep the process running smoothly.

Your digestive system has a huge role to play, and sometimes it needs a little help. Junk food, cakes and biscuits place a burden on digestion, as do not chewing food properly, eating too quickly and going overboard on booze.

A simple way to restore the balance is to nosh on probiotic and prebiotic foods that enhance the good bacteria in your gut. Think natural yoghurt, oats, asparagus, miso and tempeh if you want to keep your digestion chugging away properly.

3 tummy-loving tips

Getting your gut in shape is simpler than you think...

1 Get a daily hit of L-Glutamine (L-Glutamine 500 MG, £15.95, thenutricentre. com). This amino acid is thought to have a soothing effect on the digestive tract, helping to calm inflammation.

2 Incorporate enzyme-rich fruit such as papaya and pineapple in your diet. Papaya contains a special enzyme called papain and pineapple is full of bromelain. Both improve digestion.

3 As well as eating probiotic and prebiotic foods, boost your friendly gut flora with a supplement like Bioglan Probiotic Gastrohealth (£19.99, bioglan.co.uk).

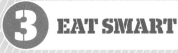
Recharge your liver

Detox your body from within to look and feel fantastic

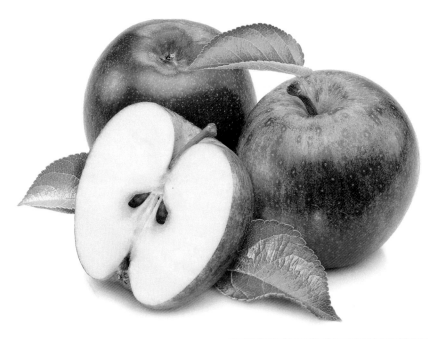

'There are simple steps that you can take to give your liver a break'

if your diet lacks roughage, bile will be shuttled back to the liver, polluting your body in the process. This has been linked to weight gain and chronic diseases.

There are simple steps that you can take to give your liver a break. Avoiding alcohol and caffeine, ditching junk food and minimising your wheat intake can all help.

Some foods also support the elimination process: fennel, artichoke and lemon are all potent cleansers and are easy to add to your diet. Squeeze lemon over salads, sip on fennel tea throughout the day and nosh on grilled artichokes as a side dish to get your liver working better.

Your liver is one of the body's most important organs. This hard-worker helps to expel potentially harmful waste from your body including excess hormones, diet nasties and alcohol. Feeling sluggish and bloated? Experiencing skin breakouts and dark circles? Or having difficulty shedding weight? These are all signs you need to show your liver a little love.

As the body's major detoxification tool, the liver pumps out waste via a substance called bile in the small intestine. Fibre is needed for this to happen effectively – so,

3 liver-loving tips

It's not just cutting things out, it's adding things in...

1 Take one tablespoon of Linwood Flaxseed with Biocultures and Vitamin D (£5.80, asda. com) daily. Simply sprinkle it in salads or stir into porridge.

2 Pop a good-quality milk thistle supplement such as Solgar Milk Thistle 100mg (£21.94, nutricentre.com). Most studies say milk thistle improves liver function.

3 Load up on fibrous fruits and veggies such as apples, pears and sweet potato. Fibre is crucially important to the liver's cleansing process, and these are tasty too!

Love your lymph

Want glowing skin and great health? Don't ignore this key system

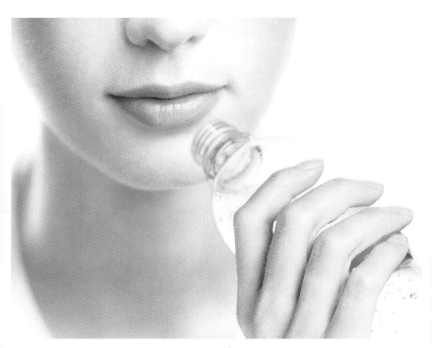

So by now you know the importance of good gut health and a well-functioning liver. However, there's another essential elimination channel in the weight-loss picture.

The lymphatic system is the body's second circulation system, and its main job is to flush out toxins via drainage ducts located in the body's tissues. The result? Improved skin firmness and elasticity, less water retention and brighter, glowing skin without a hint of orange peel.

Along with the aesthetic benefits, a happy lymphatic system equals improved

'The way this system functions plays a vital role in your health'

immunity and heart health. How? It transports nutrients in a clear fluid called lymph via a network of vessels.

The way this system functions plays a vital role in determining your overall health. Fortunately, there are a few simple steps you can take to ensure the process

runs smoothly. Eating a good diet (plenty of water flavoured with lemon juice and lots of fresh fruit), keeping active and daily body brushing all help to stimulate the detoxification process.

Doing the last of those before you shower is one of the quickest and easiest lymphatic boosters. Using a natural-fibre body brush, work long strokes from your feet upwards, brushing toward your heart. This will slough off dead cells and help to create gorgeously smooth skin!

3 lymph-loving tips

Save your skin!

1 Sip on a minimum of two litres of water every day to aid the cleansing process and stimulate lymph flow.

2 Book a lymphatic drainage massage. This gentle therapy aids detoxification, shedding excess toxins and waste.

3 Invest in a good-quality body brush, such as The Body Shop's Body Brush Round (£8, bodyshop.co.uk) – which is exfoliating without being too harsh.

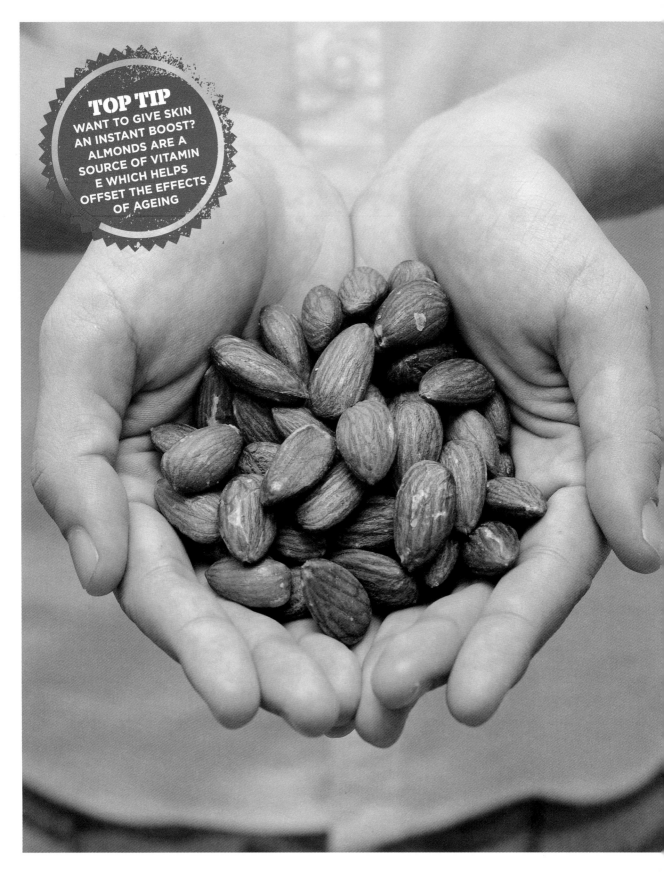

Eat up, slim down

Watch the weight melt away with these super-slimming foods

There's nothing stopping you from sculpting perfect pins and rock-hard abs. Focusing on nutritious food will help you to blast away any wobbly bits and leave you feeling fab. But if it all sounds a bit too much like hard work, you're in luck – there are some sneaky diet shortcuts that will supercharge your weight loss with minimal effort. Get ready to be a savvy eater with our guide to the best slimming foods around.

1 ALMONDS

These delicious nuts are a protein and fibre powerhouse, and will help control belly fat and keep you full between meals. Plus, they're full of magnesium, an important mineral that gives you the energy you need for a tough workout.

2 APPLES

Fruit often gets a bad rap on the diet front for its high sugar content, but as long as you pick your fruit wisely you'll reap the rewards. While some *are* high in sugar, apples are considered low GI, meaning they release their energy slowly. They're also packed with antioxidants. Stash an apple in your handbag so you always have a healthy snack on hand when those pesky cravings strike.

3 EGGS

Versatile and cheap, eggs should top your weekly shopping list. The humble egg is a fab source of protein – which you need to restore muscles after exercise – and is rich in energy-producing B vits. Whether boiled, scrambled or poached, eating eggs first thing has been shown to reduce hunger throughout the day.

> 'Focusing on nutritious food helps you to blast away wobbly bits'

4 BERRIES

Another fruity winner, dark coloured berries such as raspberries, strawberries and blueberries are chock full of health-boosting antioxidants (and strawberries – which are rich in plytonutrients – contain more vitamin C than oranges!). They also contain an impressive amount of fibre, helping your body eliminate waste so you get the flat tummy you want!

5 LEAFY GREENS

When it comes to veggies, leafy greens get a gold star. Ridiculously low in calories, but high in nutrients such as vitamin K, iron and calcium, powerhouse greens like spinach, kale and Swiss chard support the liver, keeping excess pounds at bay.

6 YOGHURT

We're not talking about the flavoured stuff here, but low-fat natural yoghurt. It helps to reduce bloating by regulating the good bacteria that lines your gut. Make sure you choose only plain, unsweetened varieties that contain live cultures for maximum gains.

7 OILY FISH

There's no doubting the slimming powers of oily fish like salmon and ▶▶

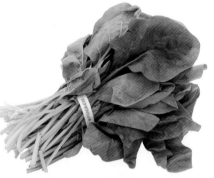

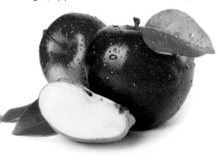

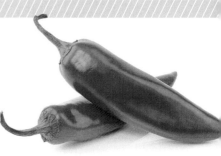

sardines. An amazing source of super-duper omega-3 fatty acids, which regulate hormones and encourage fat burn, oily fish also delivers a hit of post-workout protein. This helps repair and build lean muscle tissue, so you get the most out of every workout.

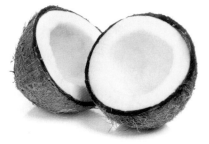

⑧ COCONUT

This tropical trooper boasts a huge array of health benefits. Coconut contains fats called medium-chain fatty acids, which help you burn fat, fast. Other studies show the exotic fruit helps to reduce tummy fat, too. The oil also doubles as a beauty essential. Use it as a body moisturiser and weekly hair mask.

⑨ CHILLI

Spicing up food with a sprinkling of fiery chilli doesn't just get your taste buds tingling, it also keeps hunger pangs at bay. Capsaicin, which is what makes chillies hot, revs up your metabolism and has been shown to fight cravings. It helps control insulin, fending off the blood

sugar spikes that cause you to store fat. Plus it raises your core body temperature, so you burn more calories at rest.

⑩ QUINOA

This underrated South American grain is high in protein and minerals, such as magnesium and calcium. Plus its high fibre content ensures you feel full, without a hint of uncomfortable bloating.

6 ways to rev it up

Take your diet to the next level with a little help from these handy supplements

1 For an inner cleanse

Detox your body from the inside out with this blend of 26 nutrients including vitamin C, iron and copper.
● Vitabiotics Wellwoman Inner Cleanse, £9.15, vitabiotics.com

2 For a healthy liver

Give a sluggish liver a kickstart with this blend of superfoods including spirulina, wheatgrass and chlorella.
● PhD Greens, £34.99, phd-supplements.com

3 For faster fat burning

This conjugated linoleic acid supplement helps to burn body fat, especially around your tum. So it's a great option to take alongside this programme.
● Solgar Tonalin CLA, £21.42, revital.co.uk

4 For a better oiled bod

This unrefined oil contains the perfect radio of omega 3, 6 and 9 to supercharge fat-burning.
● Udo's Choice Ultimate Oil Blend, £10.99, independent health food stores

5 For a speedy metabolism

Rev up your metabolism with this vitamin and mineral blend. It's packed with B vitamins, chromium and caffeine.
● Maxitone Sculptress Tablets, £9.99, maxitone.com

6 For more energy

This high-strength L-carnitine supplement helps shuttle fatty acids into the body's cells where they can be used as energy.
● Reflex L-Carnitine, £25.49, reflex-nutrition.com

TOP TIP

BORED OF PORRIDGE? PREPARE A BOWL OF QUINOA WITH NUT MILK AND FRUIT INSTEAD, FOR A NUTRITIOUS START TO THE DAY

8 savvy food swaps

Keep your weight loss on track with these easy diet solutions

A well-stocked kitchen is vital for your new healthy lifestyle, so it's time to restock your cupboards with some nourishing go-to foods. By making clever choices you'll cut calories and get a hefty dose of nutrients at the same time. Try our easy swaps and watch those excess pounds melt away.

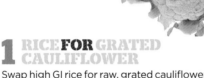

1 RICE FOR GRATED CAULIFLOWER

Swap high GI rice for raw, grated cauliflower and you'll be well on your way to meeting your body's daily vitamin C needs without any of the bloating effects of rice.

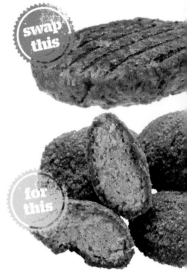

2 BEEF BURGERS FOR CHICKPEA PATTIES

For a hefty protein hit, minus the extra calories, swap minced beef for some mashed chickpeas.

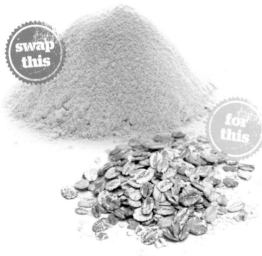

5 FLOUR FOR OATS

Ditch refined white flour for gluten-free ground oats next time you're baking and you'll get a big dose of B vitamins and none of the digestive woes that often come with regular flour.

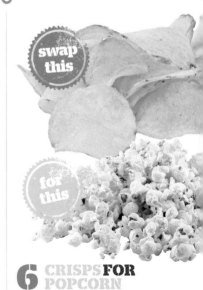

6 CRISPS FOR POPCORN

Virtually devoid of nutrients, crisps are full of fat, salt and calories. Plain popcorn is high-fibre and low-cal.

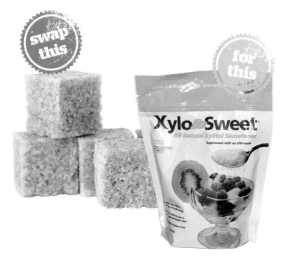

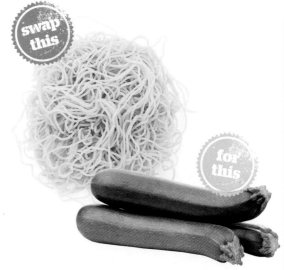

3 SUGAR **FOR** XYLITOL

If you want to enjoy the odd sweet treat, without the highs and lows that come with the regular stuff, use xylitol. It's a naturally occurring sugar that keeps your blood glucose levels stable.

4 NOODLES **FOR** COURGETTES

Spice up Asian dishes like stir-fries with courgette ribbons instead of noodles. Peel lengthways and toss into a wok with bean sprouts, peppers, spring onion, soya sauce and chilli for a carb-free dinner.

7 ICE CREAM **FOR** FROZEN FRUIT

Frozen fruit makes a far more nutritious alternative to ice cream. Purée your favourite fruit and pour the mixture into a cup. Add a lolly stick, pop it in the freezer until it's solid, and voila – a healthy homemade ice lolly!

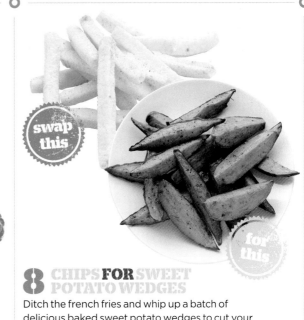

8 CHIPS **FOR** SWEET POTATO WEDGES

Ditch the french fries and whip up a batch of delicious baked sweet potato wedges to cut your calorie intake and stay fuller for longer.

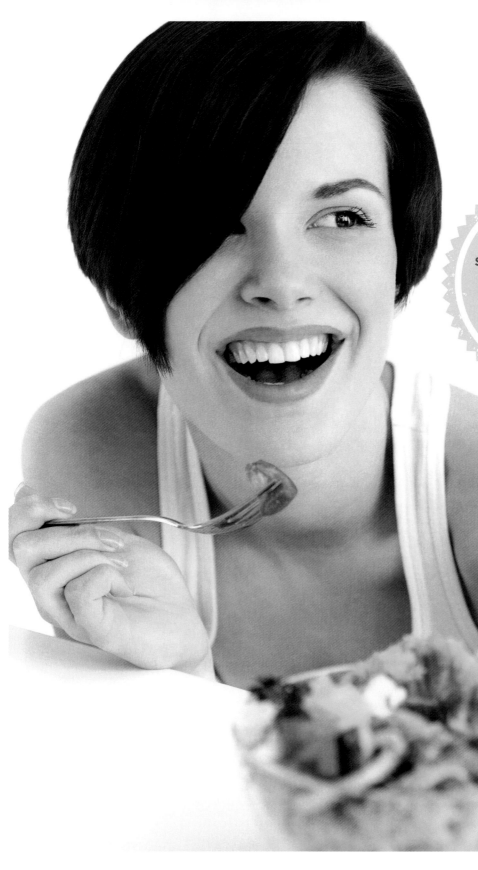

TOP TIP
DON'T DROWN
SALADS IN DRESSINGS
THAT UNDO THEIR
BENEFITS. A FRESH,
HEALTHY OPTION
IS RASPBERRY
VINAIGRETTE

The golden rules

Follow our bootcamp diet guidelines for a happier, healthier and slimmer new you

If you're sick of fad diets and slimming gimmicks you'll be pleased to hear that our four-week Drop A Dress Size bootcamp plan is designed to help you lose weight safely and keep it off for good. It works by resetting your metabolism with the right foods and fat-burning workouts. There's no deprivation involved and you're even allowed a cheat day each week.

Following this plan also helps to balance hormones that could be sabotaging your weight-loss efforts and fine-tune a sluggish digestion. We'll show you how to eat to harmonise your hormones, clean up your organs and soothe your tummy, not just to shed pounds, but to lift your mood and give you tons of energy, too.

The tailor-made exercise plans combine cardio with strength training to melt fat and leave you super toned. Plus the short and sharp workouts put your fat loss in the fast lane, leaving you time to enjoy life.

If you want this bootcamp to succeed, however, you need to commit to a few changes. Follow these 15 diet rules over the next four weeks and you'll be well on your way to your dream body.

1 LEARN TO LOVE LEMON

Start each day with a mug of hot water and lemon juice to help the liver flush impurities from your body. That's because it's an antiscorbutic: a remedy that prevents disease and assists in cleansing the system.

2 CHEW YOUR FOOD

Digestion begins in your mouth, so make sure you spend time savouring your meals. Chewing helps to release nutrients from food so that you can absorb them properly. It also stops you from overeating as it gives your brain enough time to communicate with your tum.

'Harmonise your hormones, clean your organs and soothe your tum'

3 DON'T DRINK AND EAT

Try to avoid drinking water while you eat, because it dilutes the digestive enzymes that help to break down food. Have a big glass of water about 20 minutes before you eat to help you figure out if thirst might be the cause of some of those hunger pangs. And don't drink any more until around an hour after your meal.

4 DON'T EAT LATE

Try to have your last meal of the day by 7pm to give your body ample time for

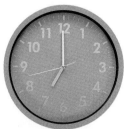

digestion before you head to bed. If you know you'll be working late, try making an extra batch of dinner the night before and taking it to work with you to ensure you stick to your early-eating routine.

5 EAT GOOD FATS

Don't be scared of fat. This macronutrient gets a bad rap, but good fats like omega 3 in oily fish, medium-chain triglycerides in coconut and monounsaturated fats from avocados actually help to rev up your fat burn.

6 READ LABELS

Look out for labels marked with hydrogenated fats and artificial sweeteners, such as aspartame, and avoid these at all costs. These products are detrimental to your diet, as they're difficult to digest and have been linked with all sorts of chronic diseases.

7 DITCH CAFFEINE

If you start the day with an espresso or think you can't function without an afternoon cappuccino, it's time to change. Caffeine picks you up only to drop you down later, so go for organic decaf varieties which are free from chemicals and substitute caffeine for energising herbal teas like rooibos and ginseng.

8 EAT FRUIT ON AN EMPTY STOMACH

Fruit, in moderation, is good for you. It's jam-packed with antioxidants and offers a convenient snack option when you're on the go. But make sure you eat fruit *before* your main meal rather than afterwards. Otherwise it can ferment in your gut, leading to bloating and indigestion.

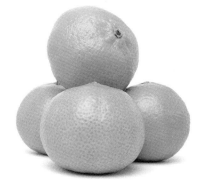

9 AVOID ALCOHOL

Alcohol is entirely devoid of nutrients and a source of empty calories. For really noticeable results, try to eliminate alcohol altogether from your diet, and if you must drink, make it a treat: allow yourself no more than one small 125ml glass of red wine each week.

10 BE A MINDFUL EATER

There are no TV dinners on this diet! Slouching on the sofa while stuffing your face will interfere with digestion, leaving you bloated and leading to overeating. Make sure you eat your meals sitting at a table, away from distractions, and sit up straight to ensure food travels through your digestive system efficiently.

11 POP A PILL

Our supplement list on page 36 will help you supercharge your weight loss

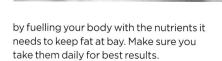

by fuelling your body with the nutrients it needs to keep fat at bay. Make sure you take them daily for best results.

12 WRITE A LIST

Map out your meals at the start of each week so you know what you'll be having in advance (there's a shopping list at the beginning of each weekly section in this book). Bring a list of ingredients with you every time you go shopping so you're not tempted to reach for junk.

13 CLEAR OUT YOUR KITCHEN

Before undertaking this diet, grab a bin bag and clear out the clutter! Donate unhealthy foods – like pre-packed cakes, biscuits and ready meals – from your fridge, freezer and cupboards to neighbours or a food bank, and get ready to restock them with healthy options.

14 AVOID THE SCALES

If you step on the scales every day and they don't move in the direction you hoped for, you're guaranteed to lose motivation. Weigh yourself no more than once a week; first thing in the morning, in your underwear, for an accurate reading. Remember: muscle weighs more than fat!

15 DRINK UP

We're talking about water here! Water helps to flush waste from your body and keeps your bowels moving nicely to reduce bloating. Sip on a minimum of two litres daily. Don't like the taste? Try adding slices of lemon and cucumber for a refreshing hit.

Pantry essentials

Overhaul your kitchen cupboards with these healthy food staples. We've given a few options for many of the food types to give you variety, but feel free to purchase just one or two if you prefer

- Wholegrain bread (wholegrain loaf, seeded loaf, wholegrain bagels, mini wholegrain pitta breads)
- Brown rice cakes
- Oatcakes
- Porridge oats
- Sugar-free muesli
- Grains (brown rice, millet, quinoa)
- Wholemeal pasta
- Sweet potatoes
- Nut milk
- Skimmed milk
- Eggs
- Houmous
- Low-fat cheese (cottage cheese, mozzarella and Cheddar cheese)
- Low-fat crème fraîche
- Lemons and limes

- Low-fat natural yoghurt
- Tofu
- Frozen berries
- Parma ham
- Smoked salmon
- Mackerel fillets
- Reduced-sugar baked beans
- Tomato purée
- Tinned chopped tomatoes
- Tinned tuna and salmon in spring water
- Good quality pre-prepared soups (lentil, bean)
- Miso soup sachets
- Dips (tomato salsa, guacamole, tzatziki)
- Tinned beans (mixed beans, butter beans, chickpeas)
- Pesto sauce

- Reduced-salt soya sauce
- Low-fat coconut milk
- Pitted olives
- Thai green and red curry pastes
- Cold-pressed oils (extra virgin olive oil, coconut oil, linseed oil)
- Balsamic vinegar
- Dried herbs (mixed herbs, parsley, rosemary, oregano, coriander)
- Fresh herbs (coriander, parsley, rosemary, basil)
- Garlic
- Spices (turmeric, chilli, curry powder, cumin, coriander)
- Desiccated coconut
- Protein powder (whey, pea, hemp)
- Raw nuts and seeds (mixed nuts, mixed seeds, chia, linseed)

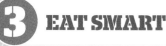

Be a cheater!

Take time off from your healthy diet and you'll reap the rewards

So you're having one of those days where you'd kill for a slice of chocolate cake and the thought of pepperoni pizza makes your mouth water? We've all been there... and the good news is that the Drop A Dress Size Diet allows you to cave in to occasional cravings. We've designated Sunday as your cheat day, when you get to indulge in your favourite meal, guilt-free!

Allowing yourself a tasty reward at the end of a long week of healthy eating doesn't equal diet failure. In fact, quite the opposite! Savouring the occasional indulgent meal helps you to stick to your diet the rest of the time, and there's even research suggesting that cheating boosts your metabolism so you burn fat faster!

As long as you follow a few key rules, giving into temptation won't hamper your diet efforts and it will give you more motivation to stick to your healthy plan.

PLAN YOUR SUNDAY SPLURGE

- Choose your cheat meal in advance to give you something to look forward to at the end of the week.
- If you're eating out, you can choose to spend your cheat meal on either the main course or dessert – not both.
- Stop eating when you feel full. Overeating will just make you feel sluggish, not satisfied.
- Chew your food properly, so you really appreciate the flavour of your favourite food instead of wolfing it down without a second thought.

CHEAT DAY GOODIES

The best way to get the most out of your reward meal is to identify what's going to hit the spot.

- If you're craving carbs...
  ...enjoy a small pizza with your favourite toppings.
- If you long for a sweet treat...
  ...indulge in two small scoops of your fave ice cream.
- If you're craving something salty...
  ...make your own BLT.
- If you're lusting after fatty food...
  ...tuck into a good-quality cheeseburger and a small serving of fries.

> 'An occasional indulgent meal helps you stick to your diet'

How to rock a cheat day

If you're indulging in a cheat meal, it's important that the rest of the day's food intake is as healthy and low-cal as possible. Here's an example of a cheat day meal plan.

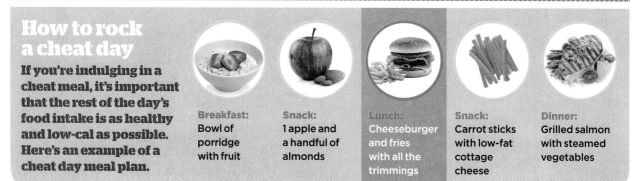

Breakfast: Bowl of porridge with fruit

Snack: 1 apple and a handful of almonds

Lunch: Cheeseburger and fries with all the trimmings

Snack: Carrot sticks with low-fat cottage cheese

Dinner: Grilled salmon with steamed vegetables

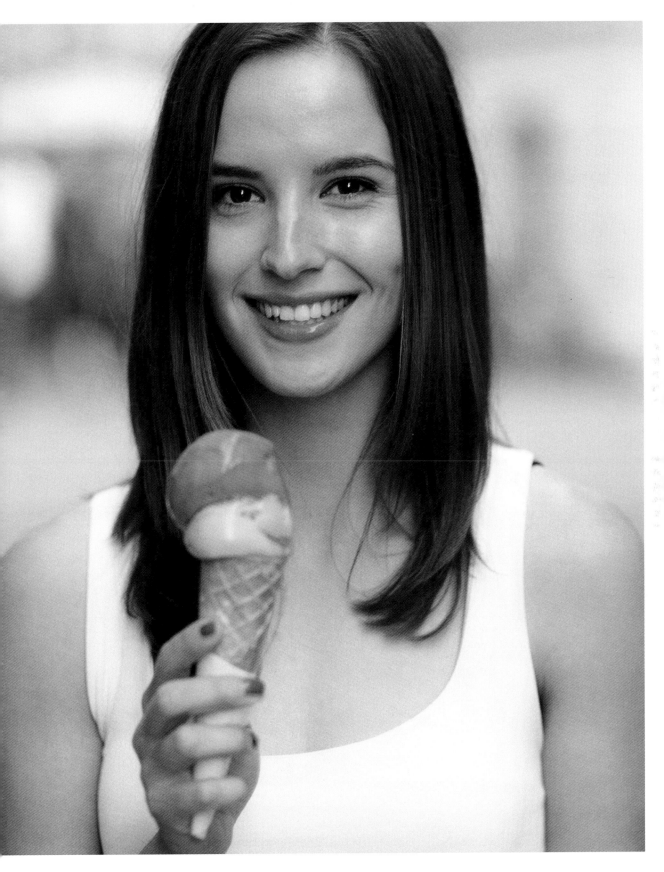

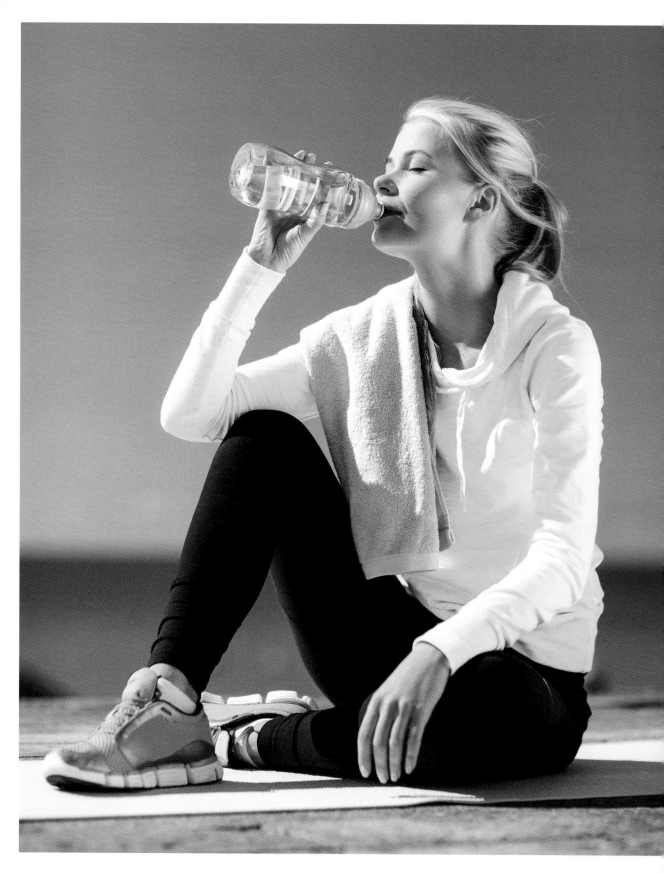

Your daily diet and workouts

Ready for a brand new you? Here's the plan you need to follow to drop that dress size in just four speedy weeks

This fat-busting, health-boosting plan is designed to help you drop a dress size in just four weeks. It's packed with low-GI, nutritious foods to keep you full, and high-intensity workouts to ramp up your weight loss. You should feel lighter and full of energy in a matter of days!

HOW IT WORKS

- Stick to the guidelines outlined on page 40 and follow each daily meal plan to the letter for the best results.
- We've designed the recipes so that they're easy to make when time is short. But they are all super-healthy and packed with nutrients and flavour.
- After exercising, have a protein bar to help repair your muscles.
- If you feel extra hungry before you're due to work out, fuel up with a small handful of raw nuts to give you the energy you need to keep going.
- If you feel hungry after following the plan for a few days, choose from the following extra snacks: a cup of miso soup, two oatcakes with nut butter or an apple and five almonds.
- Aim to have your additional snack before 6pm.

- We've designated Sunday as 'cheat day' where you can enjoy a treat meal of your choice. See our suggestions on page 44 to ensure you get the most out of your splurge without hampering your diet efforts.
- Each page also includes your workout schedule for the day. Try to stick to the plan closely to give your body a balanced combination of cardio and strength workouts. You'll find instructions for the workouts from page 84 and detailed guidelines for the cardio sessions on page 16.

'You should feel lighter and full of energy in a matter of days!'

- We've also put together handy weekly shopping lists at the start of each week and progress pages at the end to help you track your results.
- And from all your friends here at *Women's Fitness*...

Good luck!

Need to know
Follow these tips for the best chance of diet success

1 If you're eating out...
Don't despair, there are plenty of healthy options. Order a protein dish (such as fish or meat with a side salad or grilled vegetables) as a main. Ask for the sauce on the side and opt for light dressings such as vinaigrette over creamy options.

2 When you're shopping...
Buy organic whenever possible. It should be free from pesticides and fertilisers and has been shown to have higher levels of certain nutrients than non-organic food. If you can't afford to buy everything organic, prioritise dairy and meat and really wash your fruit and veg.

3 If you're vegetarian...
There are plenty of vegetarian dishes in this diet. If you don't eat meat, simply swap in veggie sources of protein such as organic tofu, pulses and eggs instead of meat.

4 Who *shouldn't* follow the diet... Although the diet is suitable for most people, there are certain people who shouldn't give it a go. If you have a medical condition, such as type 2 diabetes or heart disease, you should seek advice from your GP before beginning. Women who are pregnant or breastfeeding are also not advised to follow the diet.

Your shopping list
WEEK ONE

CHECK OUT PAGE 43 FOR A COMPLETE LIST OF PANTRY STAPLES

FRUIT
- 2 pears (or 1 packet of pears if you want to bulk buy for future weeks)
- 1 banana (or 1 bunch of bananas)
- 1 avocado
- 1 honeydew melon
- 1 apple (or 1 packet of apples)
- 2 small oranges (or 1 bag of small oranges)
- 1 small bunch of grapes

VEGETABLES
- 1 cucumber
- 1 box of cherry tomatoes
- 1 bag of stir-fried vegetables
- 2 bags of mixed salad leaves
- 1 packet of asparagus spears
- 4 red onions or (1 small packet of red onions)
- 1 bag of spinach
- 1 packet of mixed bell peppers
- 1 packet of mange tout
- 1 packet of kale
- 1 packet of new potaotes
- 1 packet of bok choy
- 1 large carrot (or 1 packet of carrots)
- 80g button mushrooms (or 1 box)

MEAT AND FISH
- 1 packet of prawns
- 1 packet of chicken breasts
- 1 packet of salmon fillets
- 1 packet of cod fillets
- 1 packet of extra lean bacon
- 1 packet of lean beef mince
- 1 packet lean pork fillets
- 1 x 170g sirloin steak

Shopping on a budget

1 Take each week's list with you to the supermarket. This will help you resist the urge to load your trolley with treats. We've categorised the list to make your shop even easier!

2 There's a variety of fruit and veg. To keep costs low and avoid waste, swap options. For example, if you have leftover rocket, use it in place of watercress.

3 Much of the fruit and veg will last more than a week. We've marked in following weeks where you may have leftovers.

4 Bulk-buy poultry, meat and fish to keep costs low. These can be easily stored in the freezer.

5 You can buy fruit and veg in individual amounts or in bigger packets to be used in the following weeks. It's up to you!

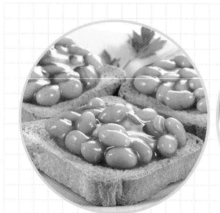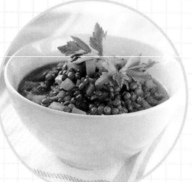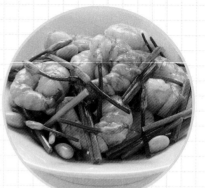

Monday

Beans on toast
Toast 1 slice of wholegrain bread and serve
with a 200g can of reduced-sugar baked beans.

2 oatcakes and 2 tablespoons of houmous.

Lentil soup
1 carton fresh, pre-prepared lentil soup served with 1 slice of rye bread.

1 pear and 3 Brazil nuts.

Prawn stir-fry
Stir-fry ½ a packet of mixed vegetables with 1 tablespoon of reduced-salt
soya sauce. Add 1 finely chopped, de-seeded chilli and 100g cooked
prawns. Garnish with the juice of ½ a lime and a sprinkling of coriander.

All levels: 25-minute workout (page 93).

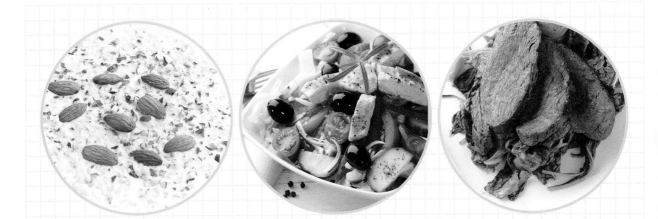

Tuesday

BREAKFAST

Nutty porridge
Cook 50g porridge oats with 70ml nut milk.
Serve sprinkled with 1 tablespoon of chia seeds or mixed seeds.

MORNING SNACK

1 banana and 4 pecan nuts.

LUNCH

Chicken salad
Combine 100g cooked chicken breast with a bag of mixed
salad leaves, 6 cherry tomatoes, 6 olives, ½ cucumber, sliced and ¼ red
onion, sliced. Drizzle with 1 tablespoon of balsamic vinegar.

AFTERNOON SNACK

2 brown rice cakes served with 2 tablespoons of low-fat cottage cheese.

DINNER

Steak with vegetables
Grill 170g sirloin steak and serve with unlimited
steamed spinach and 1 red pepper, roasted.

WORKOUT

All levels: Rest day.

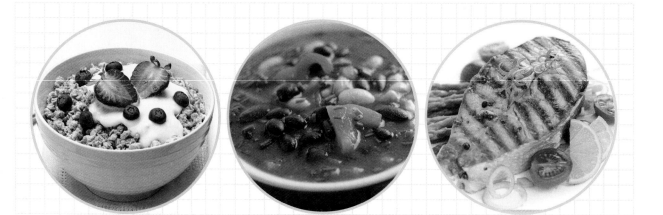

Wednesday

BREAKFAST

Muesli
30g sugar-free muesli served with 3 tablespoons low-fat yoghurt.

MORNING SNACK

50g red grapes and 7 cashew nuts.

LUNCH

Mixed bean soup
1 carton of fresh, pre-prepared mixed bean soup served
with a small wholegrain roll.

AFTERNOON SNACK

1 large carrot cut into sticks and served with 2 tablespoons of guacamole.

DINNER

Asian-style salmon with vegetables
Drizzle 1 salmon fillet with 1 tablespoon of reduced-salt soya sauce
and bake for 15 minutes. Stir-fry 50g asparagus, 1 tomato,
½ a sliced onion and 1 bok choy. Serve with lime wedge.

WORKOUT

Beginner: 15-minute cardio workout (bike).
Intermediate and advanced: 20-minute cardio workout (bike).

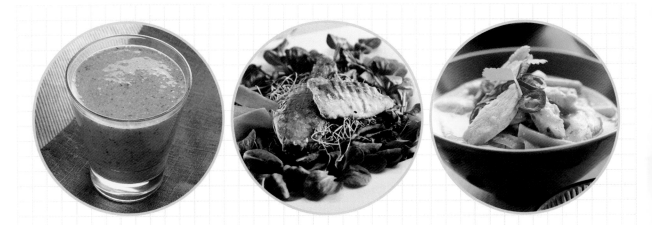

Thursday

BREAKFAST
Protein smoothie
Blend 1 scoop of whey protein with 25g mixed frozen berries and 170ml nut milk until smooth.

MORNING SNACK
1 apple and 5 almonds.

LUNCH
Mackerel salad
Combine 100g mackerel with unlimited salad leaves, 6 cherry tomatoes
and ¼ sliced red onion. Drizzle with 1 tablespoon of balsamic vinegar to serve.

AFTERNOON SNACK
2 small oranges and 2 tablespoons of pumpkin seeds.

DINNER
Thai green curry
Cut 1 chicken breast fillet into strips and fry in 1 teaspoon of coconut oil.
Add 1 teaspoon of Thai green curry paste and 50ml low-fat coconut milk. Add a handful
of mange tout peas and ½ a sliced yellow pepper. Serve with 50g quinoa, cooked.

WORKOUT
Beginner: Rest day.
Intermediate and advanced: 10-minute workout (page 85).

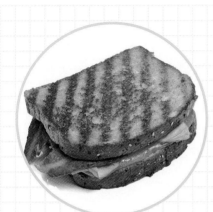
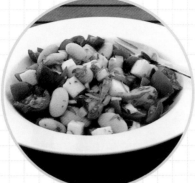
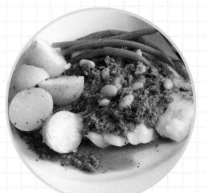

Friday

Bacon on toast
Grill 2 slices of bacon and 6 cherry tomatoes. Serve
with 1 slice of wholegrain toast.

1 pear and 5 almonds.

Butter bean salad
Combine 1 small can of butter beans with 5 cherry
tomatoes, ¼ cucumber, cubed and unlimited mixed salad leaves. Dress
with 1 tablespoon of linseed oil.

Half an avocado topped with 1 tablespoon of tomato salsa.

Pesto fish
Lightly pan-fry a 100g cod fillet and top it with 1 teaspoon of pesto sauce.
Serve it up with a green side salad and 4 boiled new potatoes.

All levels: Rest day.

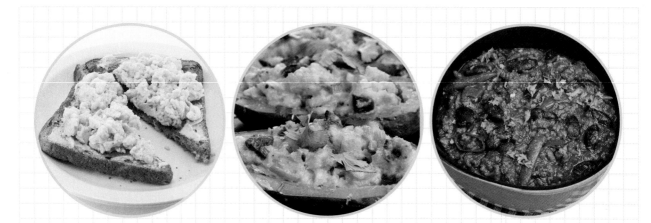

Saturday

Scrambled eggs

Scramble 2 eggs in a non-stick pan. Serve with 1 slice of seeded bread, toasted.

Half an avocado and 4 pecan nuts.

Baked sweet potato

1 baked sweet potato topped with 1 can of reduced-sugar baked beans and 15g reduced-fat Cheddar cheese.

1 cup of miso soup.

Chilli beef

Fry 1 chopped onion, 1 garlic clove and 1 chilli, chopped. Add 100g lean beef mince until browned. Add 2 tablespoons of tomato purée, 200g tin kidney beans and simmer. Serve with 50g brown rice.

All levels: Tabata workout (page 101).

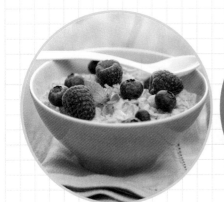

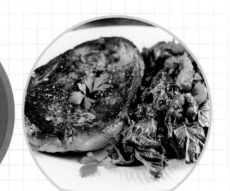

CHEAT MEAL
Enjoy a treat meal of your choice today!

Sunday

BREAKFAST
Berry porridge
Cook 50g porridge oats with 70ml nut milk. Add 2 tablespoons of mixed berries.

MORNING SNACK
1 slice of honeydew melon wrapped in 1 slice of Parma ham.

LUNCH
Cheat meal
A treat meal of your choice (see page 44).

AFTERNOON SNACK
2 oatcakes with 2 tablespoons of low-fat cottage cheese.

DINNER
Grilled pork with vegetables
Grill a 100g lean pork fillet and serve with a handful of steamed kale and 30g of sautéed mushrooms.

WORKOUT
All levels: Yoga workout (page 109).

PROGRESS REPORT

Answer the following questions to check in with how you're doing and get geared up for the week ahead

How do you feel?

What was the best part of your week?

What was the toughest part of your week?

Is there anything you could have done better/differently?

What are your goals for next week?

Your shopping list
WEEK TWO

FRUIT
- 1 punnet of strawberries
- 1 punnet of raspberries
- 1 packet of coconut chunks

VEGETABLES
- 1 courgette
- 1 cauliflower
- 1 bag of watercress
- 1 bag of rocket
- 1 bag of salad leaves

MEAT AND FISH
- 1 packet of turkey mince
- 1 packet of pork sausages
- 1 x 170g sirloin steak
- 1 can of sardines

NOTE: You may already have the following items leftover from last week's shop if you bought in bulk. If not, don't worry, we've marked the quantities you'll need below.

- 1 honeydew melon
- 1 apple
- 1 banana
- 50g red grapes

- 6 carrots
- 1 punnet of cherry tomatoes
- Half a bag of stir-fry veg
- 1 red onion
- 1 packet of spinach
- 30g button mushrooms
- 1 red and 1 yellow pepper
- 1 chicken breast
- 100g lean beef mince
- 2 slices of extra lean bacon

CHECK OUT PAGE 43 FOR A COMPLETE LIST OF PANTRY STAPLES

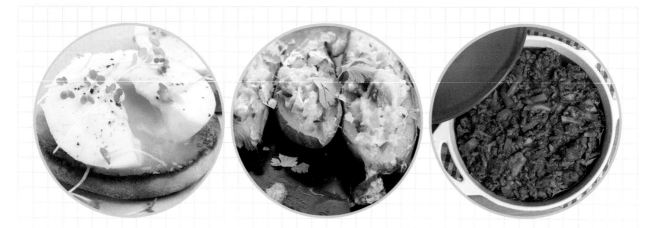

Monday

BREAKFAST
Poached eggs
Poach 2 eggs in water and serve with ½ a wholegrain bagel.

MORNING SNACK
50g chopped strawberries with 2 tablespoons of yoghurt.

LUNCH
Baked sweet potato
1 baked sweet potato served with 1 small can of tuna in spring water, drained, and 1 tablespoon of low-fat yoghurt.

AFTERNOON SNACK
2 brown rice cakes served with 2 tablespoons of guacamole.

DINNER
Carrot spaghetti with Bolognese
Cook 100g turkey mince with half a can of chopped tomatoes and 2 tablespoons of dried mixed herbs. Serve with 2 carrots peeled into ribbons.

WORKOUT
Beginner: 25-minute workout (page 93).
Intermediate and advanced: 20-minute cardio workout (running).

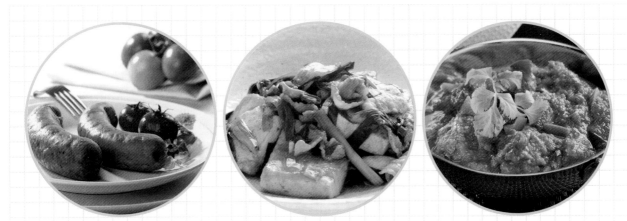

Tuesday

Sausage on toast

Grill 2 pork sausages. Serve with 3 cherry tomatoes and 1 slice of seeded bread, toasted.

1 cup of miso soup.

Tofu stir-fry

Stir-fry 100g tofu with ½ a bag of stir-fry vegetables and 1 tablespoon of reduced-salt soya sauce. Serve with 1 courgette peeled into ribbons.

30g coconut chunks and 2 tablespoons of low-fat yoghurt.

Chicken curry

Pan-fry 1 chicken breast fillet cut into strips with 1 teaspoon each of turmeric and curry powder and 2 tablespoons of low-fat yoghurt. Serve on a bed of grated cauliflower.

Beginner: Rest day.
Intermediate and advanced: 25-minute workout (page 93).

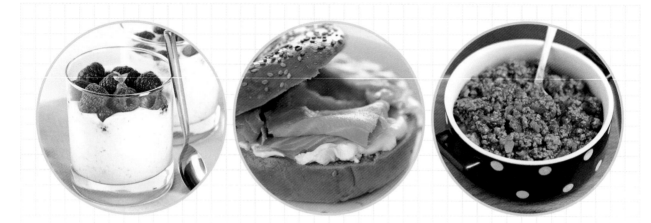

Wednesday

BREAKFAST
Berry yoghurt
1 small pot of low-fat yoghurt served with 2 tablespoons each of sunflower seeds and raspberries.

MORNING SNACK
2 oatcakes with 2 tablespoons of low-fat cottage cheese.

LUNCH
Smoked salmon bagel
Spread 2 tablespoons of low-fat crème fraîche on a wholegrain bagel.
Top with 2 strips of smoked salmon and a handful of watercress.

AFTERNOON SNACK
4 cauliflower florets served with 2 tablespoons of bean dip.

DINNER
Carrot spaghetti with Bolognese
Cook 100g turkey mince or lean beef mince with ½ a can of chopped tomatoes
and 2 tablespoons of dried mixed herbs. Serve with 2 carrots peeled into ribbons.

WORKOUT
Beginner: 15-minute cardio workout (bike).
Intermediate and advanced: Rest day.

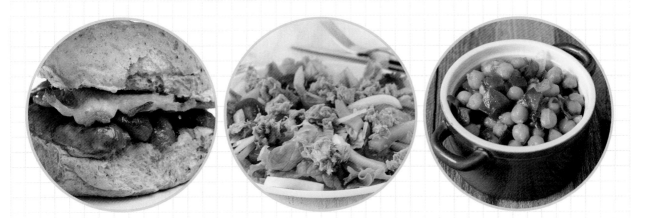

Thursday

Sausage and bacon sarnie
Grill 1 pork sausage and 1 slice of bacon.
Serve in small wholegrain roll.

2 brown rice cakes with 2 tablespoons of bean dip.

Tuna salad
Combine 1 small can of tuna in spring water, drained, with unlimited salad leaves,
6 cherry tomatoes, ¼ sliced onion and ½ a yellow pepper, sliced. Drizzle with
1 tablespoon of balsamic vinegar to serve.

1 slice of honeydew melon wrapped in 1 slice of Parma ham.

Chickpea stew
Cook ½ a can of chickpeas, drained, with ½ a can of chopped tomatoes and
1 teaspoon each of cumin and turmeric. Serve with 50g millet.

All levels: 10-minute workout (page 85).

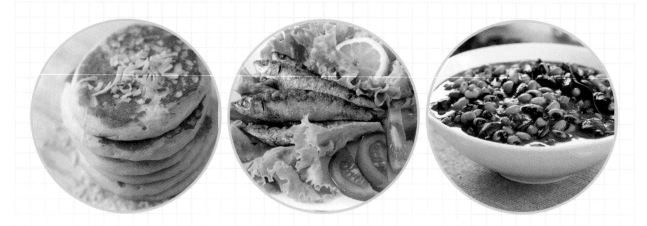

Friday

BREAKFAST
Oat pancakes
Combine 50g ground oats with 70ml skimmed milk. Ladle into a non-stick frying pan and cook on both sides. Serve with 1 tablespoon of low-fat yoghurt and 1 teaspoon of desiccated coconut.

MORNING SNACK
1 chopped apple and 5 almonds.

LUNCH
Sardine salad
Combine 100g sardines with unlimited salad leaves, 6 cherry tomatoes and ¼ sliced red onion. Drizzle with 1 tablespoon of balsamic vinegar to serve.

AFTERNOON SNACK
50g red grapes and 3 Brazil nuts.

DINNER
Bean stew
Cook ½ a can of mixed beans, drained, with ½ a can of chopped tomatoes and 1 teaspoon each of cumin and turmeric. Serve with 50g millet.

WORKOUT
Beginner: Rest day.
Intermediate and advanced: 20-minute cardio session (bike).

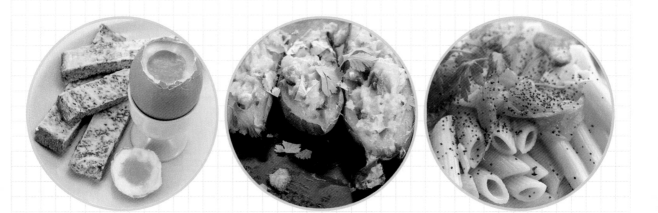

Saturday

Eggs and toast soldiers
Boil 2 eggs for 5 minutes (to ensure they are soft in the middle).
Serve with 1 slice of wholegrain toast cut into strips.

1 banana and 2 Brazil nuts.

Baked sweet potato
1 baked sweet potato topped with 1 can of reduced-sugar baked beans
and 15g reduced-fat Cheddar cheese.

1 cup of miso soup.

Salmon pasta
Cook 50g wholemeal penne pasta and toss with 100g
smoked salmon, a handful of steamed spinach and 2
tablespoons of crème fraîche.

All levels: Tabata blitz (page 101).

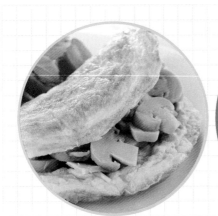

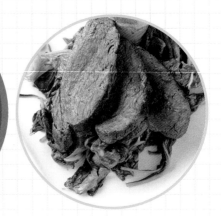

CHEAT MEAL
Enjoy a treat meal of your choice today!

Sunday

BREAKFAST
Mushroom omelette
Beat 2 eggs and add 30g sliced mushrooms. Pour into a non-stick frying pan and cook until set. Serve with ½ a toasted wholegrain bagel.

MORNING SNACK
1 scoop of whey protein blended with 200ml water.

LUNCH
Cheat meal
A treat meal of your choice (see page 44).

AFTERNOON SNACK
30g coconut pieces and 4 pecan nuts.

DINNER
Steak with vegetables
Grill 100g sirloin steak and serve with unlimited steamed spinach and 1 red pepper, roasted.

WORKOUT
All levels: Yoga workout (page 109).

PROGRESS REPORT

Answer the following questions to check in with how you're doing and get geared up for the week ahead

How do you feel?

What was the best part of your week?

What was the toughest part of your week?

Is there anything you could have done better/differently?

What are your goals for next week?

Your shopping list
WEEK THREE

FRUIT
- 1 punnet of blueberries
- 2 apples (or 1 bag of apples)
- 2 plums (or 1 punnet of plums)
- 1 peach (or 1 punnet of peaches)
- 1 banana
- 1 pear (or 1 bag of pears)
- 1 avocado

VEGETABLES
- 1 cucumber
- 1 packet of mange tout
- 1 red bell pepper and 1 yellow bell pepper (or 1 bag of mixed bell peppers)
- 1 bag of mixed stir-fry vegetables

- 2 carrots (or 1 packet of carrots)
- 1 punnet of cherry tomatoes
- 1 packet of large tomatoes
- 1 bag of mixed leaves
- 1 bag of rocket
- 1 bag of watercress
- 50g button mushrooms (or 1 box)
- 1 onion
- 1 bag of celery

MEAT AND FISH
- 1 packet prawns
- 1 sea bass fillet

OTHER
- 1 packet of pre-prepared falafel

NOTE: You may already have some of the following items leftover from the previous weeks' shop if you bought in bulk. If not, then we've marked the quantities you'll need below.

- 2 slices of extra lean bacon
- 100g lean minced beef
- 1 salmon fillet
- 1 chicken breast
- 1 packet new potatoes

TOP TIP
YOU'RE DOING REALLY WELL, SO DON'T BE TEMPTED TO STRAY FROM THE PLAN. THERE ARE LOTS OF TASTY MEALS TO COME!

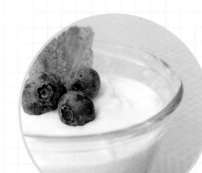
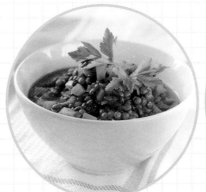
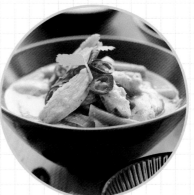

Monday

Berry yoghurt

1 small pot of low-fat yoghurt served with 2 tablespoons of blueberries and 1 tablespoon of chia or pumpkin seeds.

1 cucumber cut into sticks and served with 2 tablespoons of tzatziki.

Lentil soup

1 carton of fresh, pre-prepared lentil soup served with 1 slice of rye bread.

1 peach and 4 walnuts.

Thai green curry

Cut 1 chicken breast fillet into strips and fry in 1 teaspoon of coconut oil. Add 1 teaspoon of Thai green curry paste and 50ml low-fat coconut milk. Add a handful of mange tout and ½ a sliced yellow pepper. Serve with 50g quinoa, cooked.

Beginner: 25-minute workout (page 93).
Intermediate and advanced: 10-minute workout (page 85).

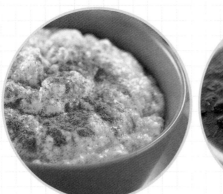 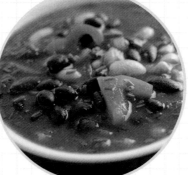 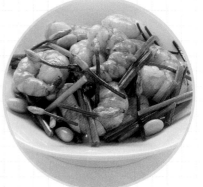

Tuesday

BREAKFAST

Cinnamon porridge
Cook 50g oats with 70ml skimmed milk. Top with 1 tablespoon of cinnamon.

MORNING SNACK

Unlimited celery cut into sticks and served with 2 tablespoons of houmous.

LUNCH

Mixed bean soup
1 carton of fresh, pre-prepared soup served with a small wholegrain roll.

AFTERNOON SNACK

1 apple and 5 almonds.

DINNER

Prawn stir-fry
Stir-fry ½ a packet of mixed vegetables with 1 tablespoon of reduced-salt soya sauce. Add 1 finely chopped, de-seeded chilli and 100g cooked prawns. Garnish with the juice of ½ a lime and a sprinkling of coriander.

WORKOUT
Beginner: 15-minute cardio workout (rower or cross-trainer).
Intermediate and advanced: 20-minute cardio workout (running).

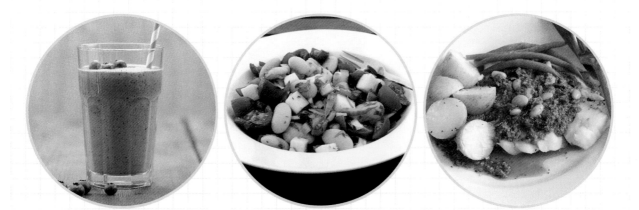

Wednesday

Blueberry smoothie
Blend 1 scoop of hemp protein with 25g mixed blueberries and 200ml nut milk until smooth.

1 slice of rye bread topped with 2 tablespoons of tomato salsa.

Butter bean salad
Combine 1 small can of butter beans with 5 cherry tomatoes, ¼ cucumber, cubed and unlimited mixed salad leaves. Dress with 1 tablespoon of linseed oil.

2 plums and 5 walnuts.

Pesto fish
Lightly pan-fry a 100g cod fillet and top it with 1 teaspoon of pesto sauce. Serve it up with a green side salad and 4 boiled new potatoes.

Beginner: 10-minute workout (page 85).
Intermediate and advanced: 25-minute workout (page 93).

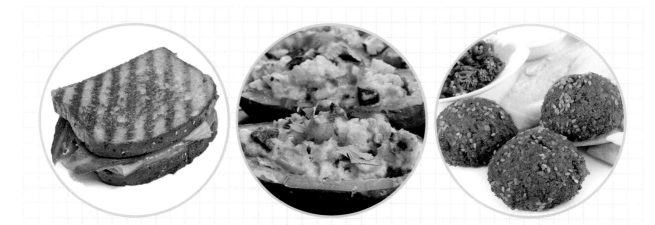

Thursday

BREAKFAST

Bacon on toast

Grill two slices of bacon and 6 cherry tomatoes. Serve with 1 slice of toasted wholegrain bread.

MORNING SNACK

1 red pepper cut into sticks and served with 2 tablespoons of low-fat yoghurt.

LUNCH

Baked sweet potato

1 baked sweet potato served with 1 small can reduced-salt baked beans and 15g low-fat Cheddar cheese.

AFTERNOON SNACK

1 peach and 7 cashew nuts.

DINNER

Mezze plate

4 falafel with 2 tablespoons of houmous and 100g tabbouleh made with parsley, chopped tomato, cucumber and lemon juice.

WORKOUT

All levels: Rest day.

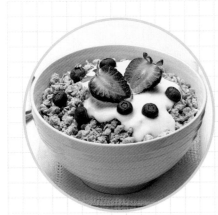
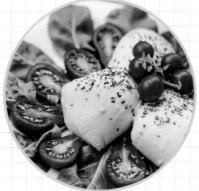
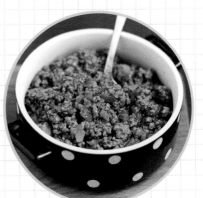

Friday

Muesli
30g sugar-free muesli served with 3 tablespoons low-fat yoghurt.

1 chopped apple and 5 almonds.

Mozzarella pitta
2 small wholemeal pitta breads filled with 100g low-fat
mozzarella, 6 cherry tomatoes, sliced and a handful of rocket.

Carrot spaghetti with Bolognese
Cook 100g turkey mince or lean beef mince with ½ a can of chopped
tomatoes and 2 tablespoons of dried mixed herbs. Serve with
2 carrots peeled into ribbons.

Beginner: 15-minute cardio workout (bike).
Intermediate and advanced: 20-minute cardio workout (bike).

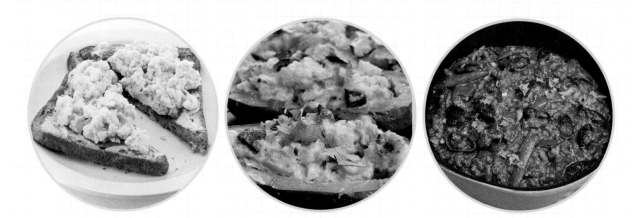

Saturday

BREAKFAST

Scrambled eggs

Scramble 2 eggs in a non-stick pan. Serve with 1 slice of seeded bread, toasted.

MORNING SNACK

Half an avocado and 4 pecan nuts.

LUNCH

Baked sweet potato

1 baked sweet potato topped with 1 can of reduced-sugar baked beans
and 15g reduced-fat Cheddar cheese.

AFTERNOON SNACK

1 cup of miso soup.

DINNER

Chilli beef

Fry 1 chopped onion, 1 garlic clove and 1 chilli, chopped. Add 100g lean beef mince until
browned. Add 2 tablespoons of tomato purée, 200g tin kidney beans and simmer.
Serve with 50g brown rice.

WORKOUT

All levels: Tabata workout (page 101).

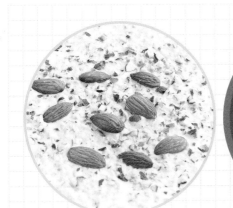

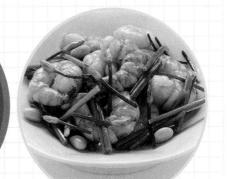

CHEAT MEAL
A treat meal
of your choice
here today!

Sunday

BREAKFAST

Nutty porridge
Cook 50g porridge oats with 70ml nut milk.
Serve with 1 tablespoon of chia or mixed seeds.

MORNING SNACK

1 banana and 4 pecan nuts.

LUNCH

Cheat meal
A treat meal of your choice (see page 44).

AFTERNOON SNACK

1 pear and 2 tablespoons of pumpkin seeds.

DINNER

Prawn stir-fry
Stir-fry ½ a packet of mixed vegetables with 1 tablespoon of reduced-salt
soya sauce. Add 1 finely chopped, de-seeded chilli and 100g cooked
prawns. Garnish with the juice of ½ a lime and a sprinkling of coriander.

WORKOUT

All levels: Yoga workout (page 109).

PROGRESS REPORT

Answer the following questions to check in with how you're doing and get geared up for the week ahead

How do you feel?

What was the best part of your week?

What was the toughest part of your week?

Is there anything you could have done better/differently?

What are your goals for next week?

Your shopping list
WEEK FOUR

FRUIT
- 1 punnet of strawberries
- 1 punnet of raspberries
- 1 small bunch of red grapes
- 1 packet of coconut chunks

VEGETABLES
- 1 punnet of cherry tomatoes
- 1 aubergine
- 1 cabbage
- 1 bag of spinach
- 1 bag of stir-fry vegetables
- 1 onion
- 1 packet asparagus spears
- 1 cucumber
- 1 cauliflower
- 1 packet of bok choy

MEAT AND FISH
- 100g lamb chops

NOTE: You may already have some of the following items leftover from previous weeks if you bought in bulk. If not, don't worry, we've marked the quantities you'll need.

- 100g turkey mince
- 2 chicken breasts
- 2 salmon fillets
- 100g prawns
- 2 plums

- 1 peach
- 25g blueberries
- 2 pears
- 1 bag of mixed leaves
- 1 yellow, 1 red, ½ green bell peppers
- 80g button mushrooms
- Handful of mange tout
- Celery sticks
- 1 large tomato
- 2 falafels

CHECK OUT PAGE 43 FOR A COMPLETE LIST OF PANTRY STAPLES

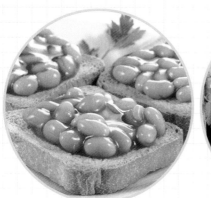
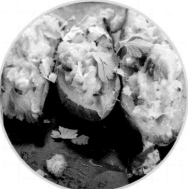
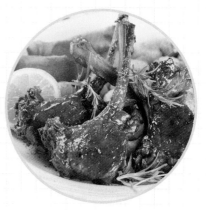

Monday

BREAKFAST
Beans on toast
Toast 1 slice of wholegrain bread and serve with
1 small 200g can of reduced-sugar baked beans.

MORNING SNACK
2 plums and 2 tablespoons of mixed nuts.

LUNCH
Baked sweet potato
1 baked sweet potato topped with a can of flaked salmon, drained, and
2 tablespoons of low-fat natural yoghurt. Serve with a green side salad.

AFTERNOON SNACK
Blend 1 scoop of pea protein with 200ml water.

DINNER
Lamb chops
Grill 100g lamb chops seasoned with rosemary, and served with steamed
cabbage and 4 grilled cherry tomatoes.

WORKOUT
Beginner: 15-minute cardio workout (rower or cross-trainer).
Intermediate and advanced: 20-minute cardio workout (running).

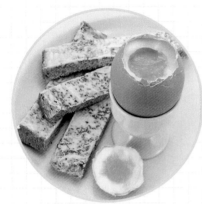
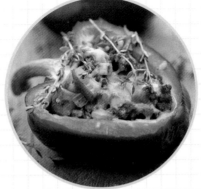
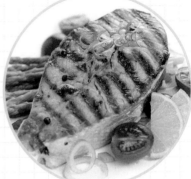

Tuesday

Eggs and toast soldiers

Boil 2 eggs for 5 minutes (to ensure they are soft in the middle).
Serve with 1 slice of wholegrain toast cut into strips.

1 peach and 4 walnuts.

Stuffed pepper

Bake 1 red pepper stuffed with 100g pan-fried turkey mince.
Serve with a green salad.

3 slices of grilled aubergine topped with 30g melted low-fat mozzarella.

Salmon and vegetables

Pan-fry 1 salmon fillet. Stir-fry 50g asparagus, 1 tomato,
½ a sliced onion and 1 bok choy. Serve with lime wedge.

Beginner: 25-minute workout (page 93).
Intermediate and advanced: 10-minute workout (page 85).

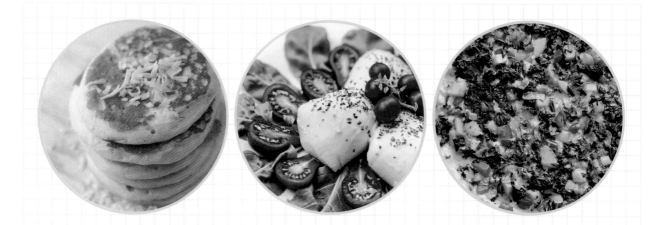

Wednesday

BREAKFAST
Oat pancakes
Combine 50g ground oats with 70ml skimmed milk. Ladle into a non-stick frying pan and cook on both sides. Serve with 1 tablespoon of low-fat yoghurt and 2 tablespoons of chopped strawberries.

MORNING SNACK
2 brown rice cakes served with 2 tablespoons of guacamole.

LUNCH
Mozzarella pitta
2 small wholemeal pitta breads filled with 100g low-fat mozzarella, 6 cherry tomatoes, sliced and a handful of rocket.

AFTERNOON SNACK
1 cup miso soup.

DINNER
Spinach and pepper omelette
Beat 2 eggs and add ½ a chopped red pepper and a handful of spinach. Ladle into a non-stick frying pan and cook.

WORKOUT
All levels: Rest day.

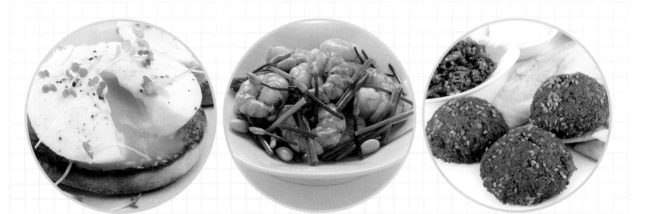

Thursday

Poached eggs
Poach two eggs in boiling water and serve with ½ a wholegrain bagel.

50g chopped strawberries with 2 tablespoons of yoghurt.

Prawn stir-fry
Stir-fry ½ a packet of mixed vegetables with 1 tablespoon of reduced-salt soya sauce.
Add 1 finely chopped, de-seeded chilli and 100g cooked prawns.
Garnish with the juice of ½ a lime and a sprinkling of coriander.

30g coconut pieces and 3 Brazil nuts.

Mezze plate
4 falafel served with 2 tablespoons of houmous and 100g tabbouleh made with
parsley, chopped tomato and cucumber and lemon juice.

Beginner: 10-minute workout (page 85).
Intermediate and advanced: 25-minute workout (page 93).

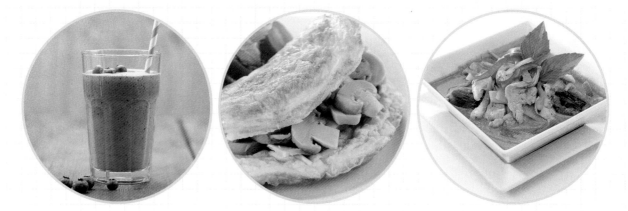

Friday

Blueberry smoothie
Blend 1 scoop of hemp protein with 25g mixed blueberries and 170ml nut milk until smooth.

1 pear and 4 walnuts.

Mushroom omelette
Beat 2 eggs and add 30g sliced mushrooms. Pour into a non-stick
frying pan and cook until set. Serve with a green side salad.

3 slices of grilled aubergine with 30g melted low-fat mozzarella.

Thai red curry
Cut 1 chicken breast fillet into strips and fry in 1 teaspoon of coconut oil. Add 1 teaspoon
of Thai red curry paste and 50ml low-fat coconut milk. Add a handful of mange tout
and ½ a sliced green pepper, sliced. Serve with 50g quinoa, cooked.

WORKOUT
Beginner: 15-minute cardio workout (bike).
Intermediate and advanced: 20-minute cardio workout (bike).

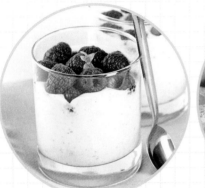
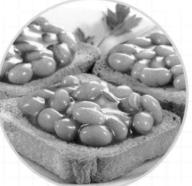
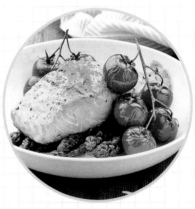

Saturday

Berry yoghurt
1 small pot low-fat yoghurt served with 2 tablespoons
each of sunflower seeds and raspberries.

Unlimited celery cut into sticks and served with
2 tablespoons of houmous.

Beans on toast
Toast 1 slice wholegrain bread and serve with
1 small 200g can of reduced-sugar baked beans.

50g red grapes and 4 pecan nuts.

Lemon salmon with vegetables
Drizzle 1 salmon fillet with 1 tablespoon of lemon juice and bake for 15 minutes.
Stir-fry 8 aspargus spears and roast 12 cherry tomatoes. Serve.

WORKOUT
All levels: Tabata blitz (page 101).

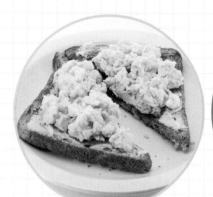

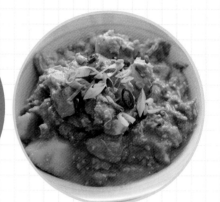

CHEAT MEAL
Enjoy a treat meal of your choice today!

Sunday

BREAKFAST
Scrambled eggs
Scramble 2 eggs in a non-stick pan.
Serve with 1 slice of seeded bread, toasted.

MORNING SNACK
1 cucumber cut into sticks and served with 2 tablespoons of houmous.

LUNCH
Cheat meal
A treat meal of your choice (see page 44).

AFTERNOON SNACK
1 pear and 4 walnuts.

DINNER
Chicken curry
Fry 1 chicken breast fillet, cut into strips, with 1 teaspoon each
of turmeric and curry powder and 2 tablespoons of low-fat yoghurt.
Serve on a bed of grated cauliflower.

WORKOUT
All levels: Yoga workout (109).

PROGRESS REPORT

Answer the following questions to check in with your progress and make a plan for maintaining your new look

How do you feel?

What were the best bits of the programme?

What were the toughest bits of the programme?

Is there anything you could have done better/differently?

If you've hit your goal, it's time to make a new one!
Write your short and long term goals below

One-month goal:

Three-month goal:

Six-month goal:

Workout handbook

**Short on time? No problem!
We've got 10-minute workouts,
25-minute fast sessions and a
Tabata blitz to ensure you've
always got time to sweat it out**

Toned in 10

This short and sweet workout will help you shed inches, fast

TOP TIP
REMEMBER TO KEEP THE INTENSITY HIGH TO SEE REAL RESULTS

If lack of time is your usual excuse for foregoing a workout, we're about to burst your bubble. Even if 10 minutes is absolutely all you can spare, it *is* enough time to squeeze in a workout that counts.

This quick blitz uses compound exercises that target all your big muscle groups to get the most out of your precious minutes. Hitting these bigger muscles will fire up your metabolism, while the short rest periods will send your heart rate soaring

– meaning you'll still benefit from your hard work long after you've hit the showers!

HOW TO DO IT

Use a weight you can manage while keeping good form for every rep, making sure that it's heavy enough to challenge you. Perform each move back to back without rest until you have completed one set of every move, then take 90 seconds' rest and repeat the circuit again.

ALL LEVELS:

2 x 10 reps each move

KIT YOU'LL NEED
- 5-20kg BARBELL
- 3-16KG KETTLEBELL

BARBELL SQUAT

Areas trained: *Legs, bottom*

Technique

- Holding a barbell across your shoulders, bend your hips and knees, pushing your bottom back until your thighs are parallel to the floor or just lower.
- Push back up through your heels and repeat the exercise for the required number of reps.

SAFETY TIP
KEEP YOUR CHEST FACING FORWARD THROUGHOUT THE EXERCISE

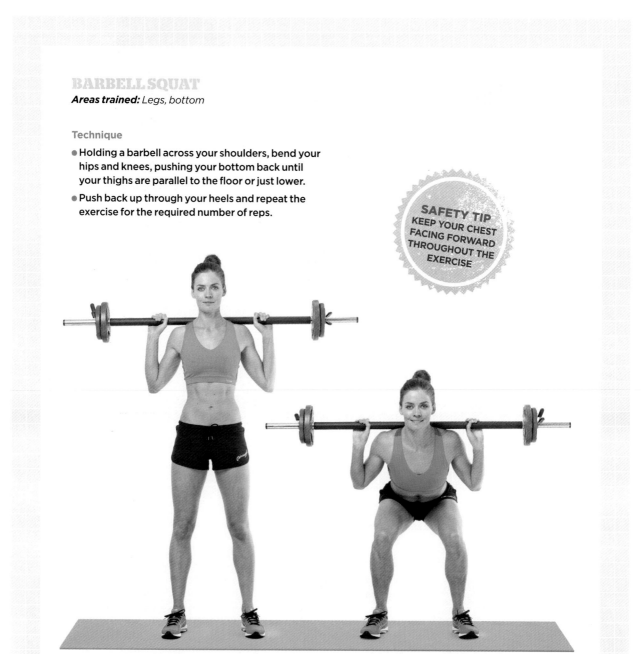

KETTLEBELL SWING

Areas trained: *Bottom, thighs, core, shoulders, back*

Technique

- Holding a kettlebell with your arms extended toward the floor, bend at your hips and knees, allowing the kettlebell to drop between your legs.
- Quickly straighten up, thrusting your hips forward and squeezing your bottom to swing the kettlebell up to around eye level.
- As the kettlebell swings back down, reverse the movement to bend at your hips and knees again, then repeat the movement in a fluid motion.

SAFETY TIP
DON'T LET YOUR UPPER BACK ARCH AT ANY POINT

CLEAN AND PRESS

Areas trained: *Legs, bottom, back, core, shoulders, rear upper arms*

Technique

- Hold a barbell in front of your thighs with your knees slightly bent.
- Bend your arms to row the barbell up to your chin.
- Drop your body below the barbell as you rotate your grip so your palms are facing up to the ceiling.
- Straighten your legs as you press the barbell toward the ceiling. Return to the start and repeat.

SAFETY TIP
TRY NOT TO HUNCH YOUR SHOULDERS AS YOU DO THE ROW

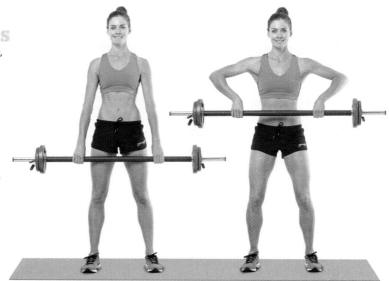

PRESS-UP

Areas trained: *Chest, rear upper arms, core*

Technique

- Start in plank position on your hands, with your body in a straight line from shoulders to toes.
- Slowly lower your chest to the floor, keeping your body straight as you do so.
- Push back up to the starting position and repeat the exercise for the required reps.

SAFETY TIP
KEEP YOUR
BACK STRAIGHT
AND DON'T HINGE
AT THE HIPS AS
YOU MOVE

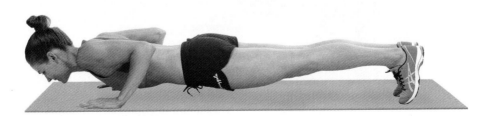

TREADMILL

Areas trained: Legs, core

Technique

- Start in plank position on your hands, with your body in a straight line from shoulders to toes.
- Jump one foot forward, keeping the rest of your body as still as possible as you do so.
- Jump it back again as you jump the other foot forward and continue fluidly to complete the set. Two leg changes equals one rep.

SAFETY TIP
KEEP YOUR HANDS DIRECTLY UNDER YOUR SHOULDERS

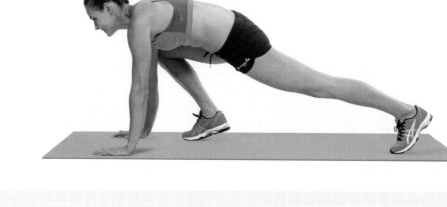

SKATER

Areas trained: *Legs, core*

Technique

- Stand balancing on your right leg.
- Jump as far to the left as possible, landing on your left leg and crossing your right leg behind it.
- Repeat on the other side and continue fluidly to complete the set. Two jumps equals one rep.

BENT-OVER ROW

Areas trained: *Upper back, front upper arms*

Technique

- Start holding a barbell with your arms extended toward the floor, bend your legs and hinge at your hips to lean your upper body forward slightly.
- Row the barbell up to your ribs.
- Lower to the starting position and repeat.

SAFETY TIP
KEEP YOUR
SHOULDERS BACK
THROUGHOUT THE
MOVEMENT

Total body blitz

Yes, you can get a full-body workout in less than half an hour. Here's how to do it...

Got half an hour? This workout will get your body firing with five minutes to spare! In just 25 minutes, you can give your entire body a fat-burning blitz.

The moves in this workout really pack a punch – they work the bigger muscle groups to help you burn fat, and they isolate trouble spots like your tummy, shoulders and bottom to sculpt a sexy physique. The amount of work you'll get done in 25 minutes might not be huge, but keeping your intensity high will ensure big results. Ready, set, go!

HOW TO DO IT

Make sure that for each move, you opt for a weight that gives you a real challenge, while still allowing you to complete the exercise with good form. Perform the moves back to back without any rest, then take a 90-second break. Complete the circuit again two more times, taking 90 seconds of rest between each circuit.

ALL LEVELS:

4 x 10-15 reps each move

KIT YOU'LL NEED
● 5-25kg BARBELL
● 2 X 2-6KG KETTLEBELL

STRAIGHT-LEG DEADLIFT

Areas trained: Bottom, rear thighs, calves, back

Technique

- Keeping a slight bend in your knees, hold the barbell close to your thighs.
- Hinge at your hips and lower your upper body until the barbell reaches the middle of your shins.
- Push your heels into the floor and straighten up, to lift the barbell, raising your upper body.

SAFETY TIP
KEEP YOUR SHOULDERS BACK AND YOUR GAZE FORWARD

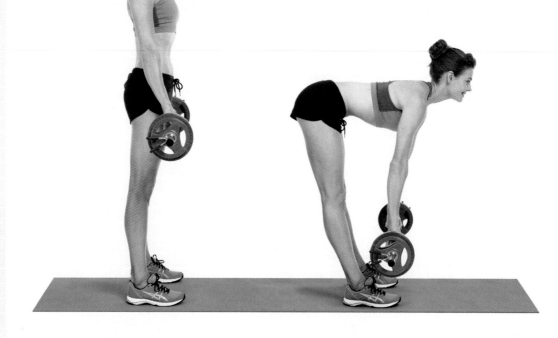

GOOD MORNING

Areas trained: *Back, rear thighs, calves, bottom*

Technique

- Hold a barbell behind your head with both hands. Let the barbell rest on the top of your shoulders.
- Keeping your back straight and knees soft, bend at your hips and push your bottom back until your upper body is parallel to the ground.
- Rise back to the starting position and repeat.

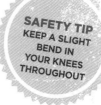

SAFETY TIP
KEEP A SLIGHT BEND IN YOUR KNEES THROUGHOUT

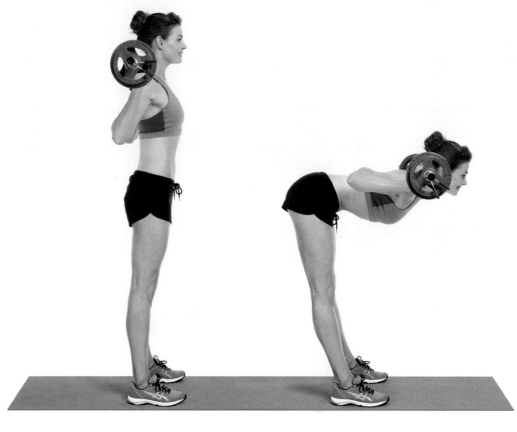

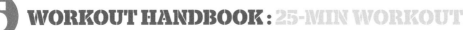

SINGLE-LEG BRIDGE

Areas trained: *Bottom, rear thighs*

Technique

- Lie on the floor with your arms by your sides, one foot close to your bottom and the other raised at a right angle toward the ceiling.
- Push up through your heel and lift your hips off the floor, as high as possible.
- Lower to the floor and repeat. Complete one set on each leg before moving on.

SAFETY TIP
RELAX YOUR NECK AND SHOULDERS

NARROW PRESS-UP

Areas trained: *Rear upper arms, shoulders, core*

Technique

- Start in plank position with hands directly under shoulders and your body in a straight line.
- Bend your arms to slowly lower your chest to the floor, keeping your upper arms close to your sides and your body in a straight line.
- Push back up to the starting position and repeat.

SAFETY TIP
MAKE SURE YOUR ELBOWS MOVE BACK, NOT OUT TO THE SIDES

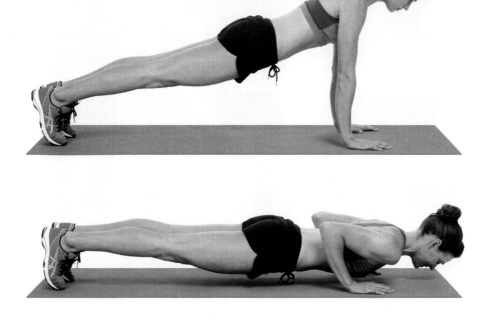

CURL AND PRESS

Areas trained: Front upper arms, shoulders

Technique

- Hold a dumbbell in each hand with your arms by your sides, palms facing forward.
- Keeping your arms close to your body, curl the dumbbells up to your shoulders, then push them up towards the ceiling, rotating your hands so your palms face forward.
- Lower the weights and repeat the exercise.

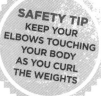

SAFETY TIP
KEEP YOUR ELBOWS TOUCHING YOUR BODY AS YOU CURL THE WEIGHTS

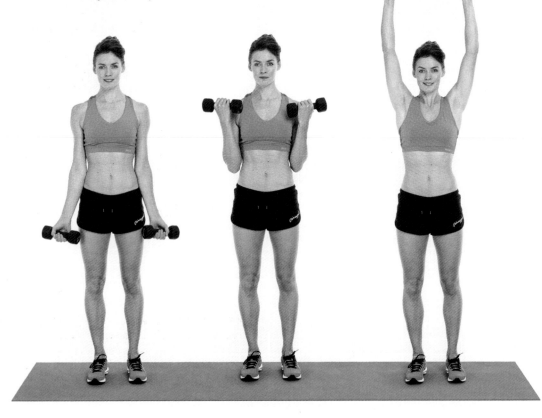

TOE TOUCH

Area trained: *Stomach*

Technique

- Lie on the floor with your feet raised at a 90-degree angle, toward the ceiling.
- Crunch up to touch your toes with your hands.
- Lower to the floor and repeat.

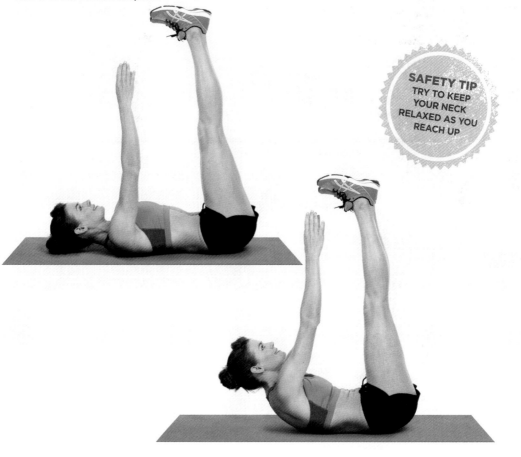

SAFETY TIP
TRY TO KEEP YOUR NECK RELAXED AS YOU REACH UP

PLANK TRANSFER

Areas trained: *Core, shoulders*

Technique

- Start in plank position with your hands under your shoulders and your body in a straight line.
- Lower your weight onto your right forearm, then your left forearm.
- Then rise on to your right hand, then your left hand.
- Keep repeating this movement, then change direction with each set.

SAFETY TIP
KEEP YOUR BODY AS STRAIGHT AS POSSIBLE, AND DON'T TILT FROM SIDE TO SIDE

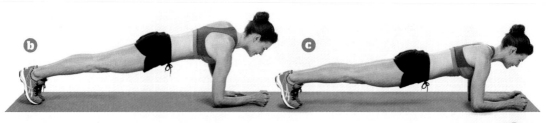

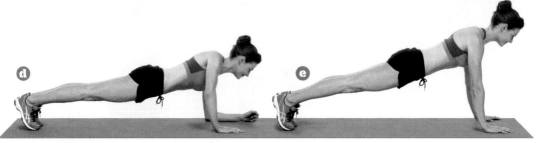

Fast and furious!

Flab to fab in four minutes flat? Yes, you can!

Four minutes. That's all you need to get fit and fight fat. Don't believe us? The Tabata Protocol, named after Japanese scientist Izumi Tabata, is based on his research with male college athletes. He found that when the guys did seven or eight blocks of 20-second sprints separated by 10-second rests, five days a week for six weeks, they boosted their aerobic fitness a whopping 14 per cent. So, when it comes to fitness, less is more.

But there is a catch. Since you're only working for 20 seconds at a time, you need to be going hell for leather! This is the ultimate version of high-intensity interval training, hitting resistance *and* cardio in one quick blitz – it's a short workout, so make every second count.

HOW TO DO IT

Choose four exercises from the following pages, make sure you target your whole body. Perform each exercise for 20 seconds and take a 10-second rest between each move. When you've completed 20 seconds of each exercise once, do all four moves again. You should be working at the highest intensity you can manage during those 20-second blocks. And that's it! Four minutes, done.

Already super fit? Repeat your circuit again for an even tougher challenge! ▶▶

KIT YOU'LL NEED
● 2 X 2-8KG DUMBBELLS

JUMPING LUNGE

Areas trained: Legs, bottom

Technique

- With one foot placed a large stride in front of the other, bend both legs to about 90 degrees until the back knee is just above the ground.

- From here, push up on the balls of your feet into a jump to switch your feet over. Land with both knees at 90 degrees again, with the opposite foot in front.

- Alternate continuously for 20 seconds.

SAFETY TIP
MAKE SURE YOUR BACK KNEE IS DIRECTLY UNDER YOUR HIP AT THE BOTTOM OF THE MOVE

JUMPING SQUAT

Areas trained: Legs, bottom

Technique

- Stand with your feet hip-width apart. Bend at your hips and knees to lower your bottom toward the floor, pushing it back as you do so.
- From this squat position, push through your legs to jump up as high as you possibly can.
- Land softly, with bent knees, and repeat the exercise for the full 20 seconds.

SAFETY TIP
KEEP YOUR HEELS FIRMLY PLANTED ON THE GROUND UNTIL YOU JUMP

BURPEE

Areas trained: *Legs, bottom, core, shoulders*

Technique

- Begin crouching, with your hands resting on the floor in front of you. Then jump your feet back into plank position.
- Jump back into a crouched position, then jump up as high as you possibly can.
- Land softly back in the crouched position and repeat for 20 seconds.

SAFETY TIP
KEEP YOUR CORE ENGAGED AS YOU JUMP YOUR FEET BACK

ALTERNATE SHOULDER PRESS

Areas trained: Shoulders, rear upper arms

Technique
- Hold a small dumbbell in each hand, just in front of your shoulders.
- Push one dumbbell straight up, toward the ceiling.
- As you lower it back to your shoulder, push the other dumbbell up to the ceiling.
- Alternate arms continuously.

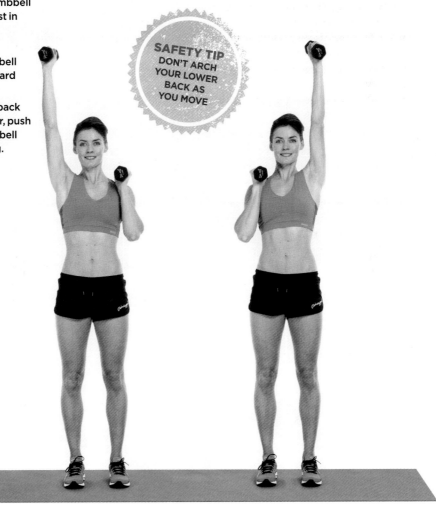

SAFETY TIP
DON'T ARCH YOUR LOWER BACK AS YOU MOVE

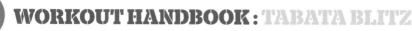

PRESS-UP RENEGADE ROW

Areas trained: *Chest, upper arms, upper back, core*

Technique

- Start in plank position holding a dumbbell in each hand, directly below your shoulders.
- Lower your chest to the floor, keeping your body straight, then push back up.
- Row one dumbbell up to your side, then lower it to the floor again.
- Bend your arms to lower your chest to the floor again, then push back up.
- Row the other dumbbell up to your side, then lower it to the floor. Repeat for 20 seconds.

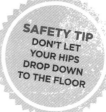

SAFETY TIP
DON'T LET
YOUR HIPS
DROP DOWN
TO THE FLOOR

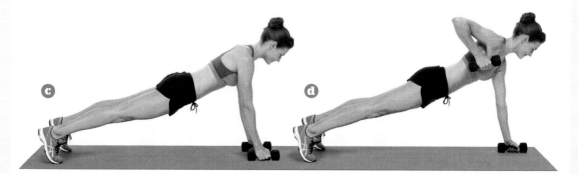

PLANK JACK

Areas trained: *Core, shoulders*

Technique

- Start in plank position, resting on your forearms with your feet together.
- Without moving your hips up or down, jump your feet apart.
- Jump your feet back to the starting position and repeat the movement for 20 seconds.

SAFETY TIP
KEEP YOUR CORE
ENGAGED AS
YOU JUMP

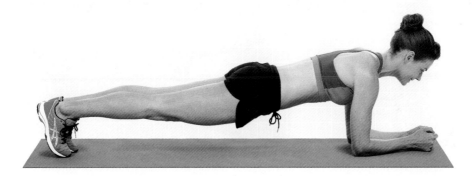

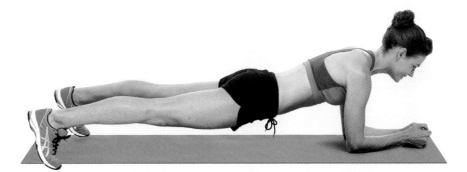

BICYCLE CRUNCH

Area trained: Stomach

Technique

- Lie on the floor with your legs and shoulders raised just a few inches off the ground.
- Keep your left leg straight and bring your right knee and your left elbow together as you rotate your upper body toward the leg.
- Return to the start and bring your left knee and right elbow together. Continue this movement fluidly for 20 seconds.

SAFETY TIP
KEEP YOUR LOWER BACK IN CONTACT WITH THE FLOOR THROUGHOUT

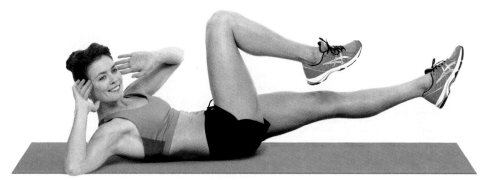

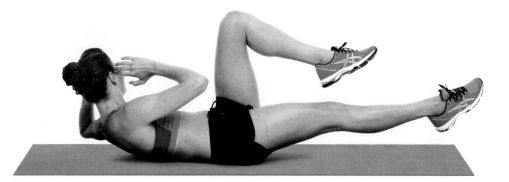

Sunday sessions

Treat your body to a day of active rest with this soothing yoga sequence

Allowing your body to unwind and recover from daily stress, work and exercise is vital for your health and your weight-loss goals. If you don't take time to defuse, stress levels can encourage your body to cling on to stubborn fat, so it really is an important part of the fat-burning puzzle.

Practising yoga helps blitz stress and improve your lymphatic system, draining toxins that could cause fat storage and cellulite. It'll also stretch out your body, soothing muscles you've worked through the week.

Doing this yoga sequence means your Sundays in the *Drop A Dress Size* programme act as an active recovery day. Your body will still be working, but in a way that aids your rest and recovery.

HOW TO DO IT

Perform each position one after the other, holding each pose for the allocated time or number of breaths. ▶▶

KIT YOU'LL NEED
- YOGA MAT
- BLOCK (OPTIONAL)

DOWNWARD DOG

What it does: *Lengthens the spine, elongates key muscles in the back, arms and shoulders, lengthens hamstrings and the Achilles tendons*

Technique

- Begin in child's pose; on your knees, with your bottom resting on your feet, your arms stretched out in front of you and your forehead resting gently on the floor.
- Check your feet are hip-width apart; your hands shoulder-width apart. Curls your toes under, inhale and press into your palms and fingers, raising your knees off the mat.
- Exhale and begin to straighten your legs, allowing your heels to drop towards the mat. This provides a stable base so you can draw and lengthen your spine towards the space between your hands.
- Ensure your spine is not rounded but elongated, as well as ensuring your shoulders do not compress or hunch up. Hold for 5 to 10 breaths.

COBRA POSE

What it does: *Opens the chest, stabilises the shoulders, strengthens the back, arms and legs, stretches the areas involved with breathing*

Technique

- Inhale and move forward into plank position, drawing your shoulders over your wrists. Then bend your arms to lower your body to the mat.
- Put your palms slightly in front of your shoulders. Raise your upper body up, keeping your hips on the floor.
- If you can, extend your arms and raise your chin. Press your pubic bone into the mat and extend your legs back, lengthening the front of your thighs away from your hips and pressing your feet into the mat.
- Keep your legs together to release the lower part of your back, or deepen the sensation by drawing your legs apart.
- Slowly draw your chest forward to engage your back muscles. Beginners should keep your arms bent and allow your lower ribs to rest on the mat so that your chest is lowered slightly.
- If you're an experienced yogi, arch your neck and lift your chin, opening your throat, but take care not to jam your neck.
- Hold for 5 to 20 breaths, then lower your chest to the floor.
- Slowly move back into downward dog, then step your feet forward between your hands, keeping your palms flat on the mat. You may need to bend your knees.

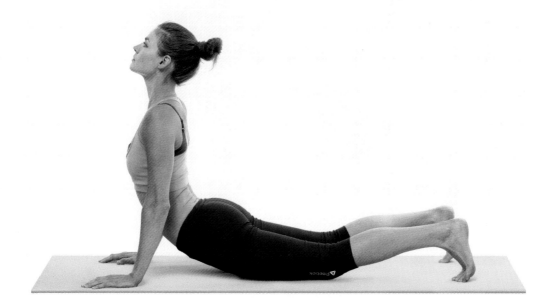

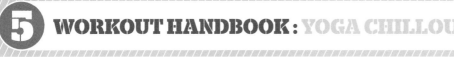

STANDING FORWARD BEND

What it does: *Extends the spine, stretches and opens the pelvis and lower back muscles, stretches the legs and strengthens feet*

Technique

- Stand with your feet together or hip-width apart.
- Fold forward, drawing your sit bones up, lengthening them away from your heels. Use gravity to help draw your chest toward your thighs. Gently draw up with your knees and thigh muscles and keep your legs strong.

- As a variation, you can interlace your fingers behind your back and gently draw your arms overhead. Allow your shoulder blades to move away from each other and your armpits to move toward the floor. Hold for 5 to 15 breaths.
- Release your arms and roll up slowly along your spinal column.

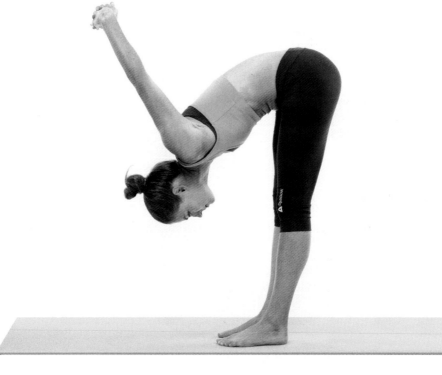

EXTENDED TRIANGLE POSE

What it does: *Extends the spine, opens the pelvis and chest, increases hip mobility, strengthens calf muscles and front thighs, and strengthens the arms*

Technique

- Face the side of your mat and step your feet out wide, with your right foot pointing forwards your left foot turned to face the side of your mat. Extend your arms out sideways, ensuring they don't rise above your shoulders. Keep your spine long and your tailbone tucked in.
- Lower your left hand to your shin, to a block (if you're a beginner) or to the floor (if you're experienced). Ensure both legs remain straight, gently drawing up with your thigh muscles and knees. Keep your hips and shoulders open.
- Inhale and slowly raise your right arm to the ceiling. If you can do so comfortably, turn your gaze to the ceiling. If this is painful, keep looking forward so as not to strain your neck.
- Hold for 5 to 15 breaths. Inhale and come back up to standing, then repeat with your feet facing the opposite way.
- Bring your feet together and fold forward. Place your hands on the mat and step back into downward dog.

BOW POSE

What it does: *Extends the spine, opens the hip flexors, strengthens the legs and firms the bottom*

Technique

- Drop to your knees, cross your ankles behind you, roll over your feet and extend your legs out in front of you. Lie on your back, then roll onto your front. Allow the muscles on either side of your spine to settle.

- Bend your knees, keeping them as wide as your hips, and flex your feet. Hold your ankles or the backs of your feet, keeping your thighs parallel.
- Press your ankles back and your tailbone toward the mat.

- Inhale and lift your head and shoulders off the mat. As you exhale, press your shins into the palms of your hands and lift your torso and legs up.
- Hold for 5 to 15 breaths.
- Lower and release your ankles.

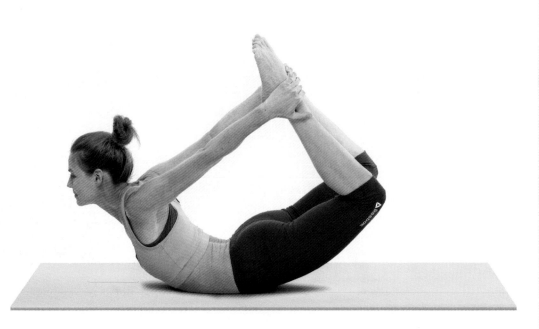

BRIDGE POSE

What it does: *Extends the hips and rear thighs, releases tension and opens the shoulders*

Technique

- Roll over to lie on your back with your knees bent and your feet flat, a few inches from your bottom. Place your arms by your sides.
- Inhale and gently tip your hips upward. Slowly exhale and press into your feet to lift up your hips and rest on your shoulders.
- Interlace your fingers behind your back and press your arms and hands into the mat to stabilise and lift your hips higher. Alternatively, place your hands at your trouser line and support your lower back with your palms.
- If you struggle with this pose, place a block under your hips in the centre, with its narrow edge in the same direction as your spine.
- Hold for 10 to 30 breaths.
- Lower your body by rolling down through your spinal column, vertebrae by vertebrae.
- Remove the block if you used one.

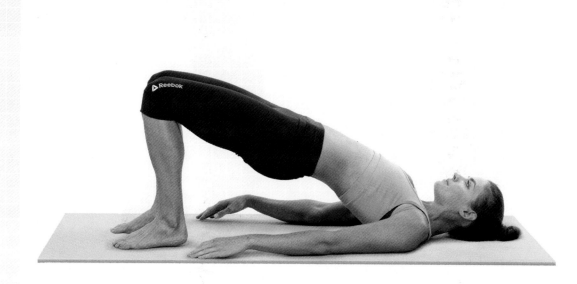

SHOULDER STAND

What it does: *Lengthens the spine and relieves tension in the head, shoulders and neck.*

Technique

- Remain on your back and lift your legs toward the ceiling, keeping your arms on the floor for stability.
- Slowly reach your legs up higher towards the ceiling by lifting your hips off the floor. Support your lower back with your hands if necessary. Keep your neck lengthened to ensure that you're not putting undue stress on your neck .

- Hold for 15 to 30 breaths.
- Slowly roll down through the spinal column to bring your feet back to the mat.

SAFETY TIP
SKIP THIS POSE
IF YOU HAVE ANY
LOWER BACK
PROBLEMS

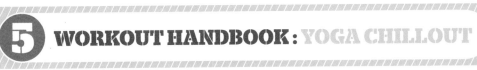

Stretch it out

Take the time to cool down after your intense bootcamp workouts for better body gains

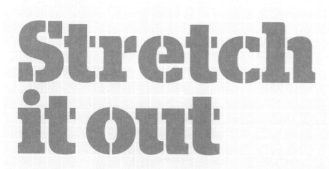

Whether you've pushed yourself to the limit for four minutes or 40, it's tempting to simply collapse in a heap when your workout is done. But, cooling down is a must if you want to keep your body injury-free, reduce muscle aches and maximise the benefits of the exercise you've just done.

Cooling down post-workout will help your body repair and recover in time for your next session so you can keep going strong for the full four weeks. When your heart rate comes down, it's important to do some gentle stretches while your muscles are still warm enough to feel the benefit. So, if you're keen to make the most of this bootcamp, don't skip the cool-down. Just grab a mat and turn on those chill out tunes!

HOW TO DO IT

Hold each stretch for 20-30 seconds each side and move straight onto the next. ▶▶

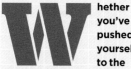

TOP TIP
SORE MUSCLES CAN PUT YOU OFF YOUR NEXT WORKOUT, SO ALWAYS STRETCH TO ENSURE YOU'RE READY FOR TOMORROW

LYING GLUTE STRETCH

Areas trained: Bottom, hips

Technique

- Lie on the floor on your back. Bend your left leg, turn the knee outwards and place your ankle on top of your right thigh.
- Lying on your back, grasp your right thigh and gently pull it towards you.
- Change sides to stretch the other leg.

SAFETY TIP
GENTLY PUSH YOUR CROSSED LEG WITH YOUR ELBOW TO INCREASE THE STRETCH

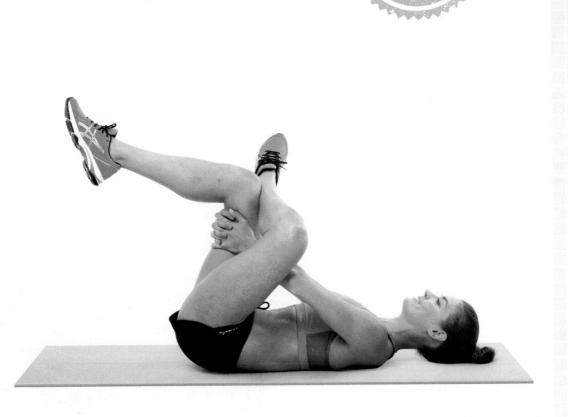

LYING HAMSTRING STRETCH

Areas trained: *Rear thighs, calves*

Technique

- Lie on your back on a mat and place your left leg flat on the floor.
- Keeping your right leg straight, grasp the back of your thigh and pull it toward you. Flex your foot to stretch your calf muscle.
- Change sides to stretch the other leg.

SAFETY TIP
ONLY GO AS FAR AS IS COMFORTABLE AND TRY TO KEEP YOUR RAISED LEG STRAIGHT

KNEELING HIP FLEXOR STRETCH

Areas trained: *Front thighs, hips*

Technique

- Kneel on your left leg and place your right foot flat on the floor in front of you.
- Lean forward and push down into your hips.
- Change sides to stretch the other hip flexor.

SAFETY TIP
KEEP YOU UPPER BODY RAISED, DON'T COLLAPSE OVER THE FRONT LEG

CHILD'S POSE

Area trained: *Back*

Technique

- Begin kneeling on the floor, then sit back on your heels and lower your upper body to the floor.
- Rest your forehead on the floor and reach your arms forward.

SAFETY TIP
SPREAD YOUR KNEES TO MAKE THIS MORE COMFORTABLE

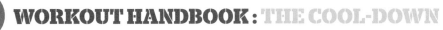

SHOULDER STRETCH

Area trained: *Shoulders*

Technique

- Bring one arm across the front of your body.
- Use the opposite arm to pull it close to your body.
- Change sides to stretch the other shoulder.

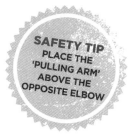

SAFETY TIP
PLACE THE 'PULLING ARM' ABOVE THE OPPOSITE ELBOW

TRICEP STRETCH

Area trained: *Rear upper arms*

Technique

- Point your elbow to the ceiling and use the opposite arm to pull it down and across to the side.
- Change sides to stretch the other tricep.

SAFETY TIP
KEEP YOUR HEAD
FACING FORWARD
RATHER THAN
DOWN

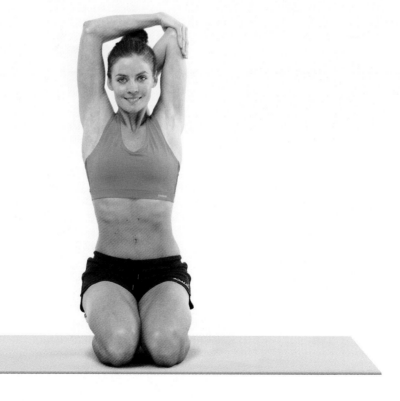

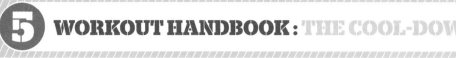

CHEST STRETCH

Areas trained: *Chest, shoulders*

Technique

- Place both hands on your lower back and gently try to bring your elbows toward each other behind your back until you feel the stretch in your chest.

SAFETY TIP
ONLY MOVE YOUR ARMS AS FAR BACK AS IS COMFORTABLE

Make your results last

A honed, toned bod isn't just for now. There's always a great excuse to slip on your LBD! So don't let your hard work go to waste: stay motivated with these helpful top tips

Dress to impress

Bootcamp: complete! Now's the time to flaunt your assets in a frock made for your figure

It's time to start showing off that hard-earned hot bod! Whether you're a bootylicious babe or a long-and-lean machine, we've got a dress to give you the 'wow' factor. After all, you've just dropped a dress size – what better excuse to go shopping for a new wardrobe?

1 CURVY QUEEN

Your best bits: A slim waist, curvy bum and ample chest.
The right frock: If you've got it, flaunt it, right? You want to show off your slim waist and flatter your killer curves, so a dress that draws attention to your middle is a good bet. Opt for something fairly snug as this will emphasise your hourglass shape and nip you in at the waist. If you're not particularly tall, a long-line dress will elongate your figure.

Hit the shops

Reiss and Whistles are a good bet for long-line dresses, but your best option is French Connection. It does a range of great-fitting bandage-style dresses that will give you that va-va-voom look.

2 LONG AND LEAN

Your best bits: A long, slim and athletic figure.

The right frock: You can get away with most styles and a lot of pattern. But to create more definition around your waist, go for a dress with detail around the middle: a belt, a sheer panel or a peplum.

Hit the shops

Topshop has great options and, with your new athletic figure, you can experiment with some of its daring styles. Or go for an all-over pattern with a belt for real impact!

3 GREAT GIRLS

Your best bits: You've got a great bust and a petite figure.
The right frock: A dress that's fitted over your breasts and nips in at the waist is essential to avoid drowning your shape in a tent-like ensemble. The key is to balance your top half: think a detailed or voluminous skirt, teamed with a plain top.

Hit the shops

Asos has a great range of dresses, so you're bound to find something that fits the bill! If in doubt, go for an attention-grabbing skirt from Zara and team with a simple top.

"It's time to start showing off that new hod bod!"

4 TUMMY TROUBLE

Your best bits: You've got lithe limbs, but a shy tummy.

The right frock: If you've got great legs and toned arms, get them out! A high hemline and strappy or short sleeves in a loose style are perfect if you'd rather not display your tummy to the waiting world. A short shift that hangs from the shoulders, or a loose frock with a hidden waist gathering will keep you feeling both sexy and comfortable.

Hit the shops

Zara is a great option if you're conscious about your tummy – it stocks lots of smock styles and loose fits in sophisticated designs.

5 BOOTYLICIOUS BABE

Your best bits: You've got a great bum and muscly legs.

The right frock: A darker colour on your bottom half is really flattering, but don't be tempted to hide your curves under swathes of fabric. Something tight will show off your great rear, especially if you're sporting a petite waist. Go for a dress that's detailed or patterned on the top, preferably with a bit of volume to balance out your ample bum.

Hit the shops

River Island has some great options with pretty, blousy and patterned top halves and black fitted bottom halves. It's definitely a winner in our book!

Stay fit for life

Make these bootcamp rules a habit to keep your best body looking and feeling good

1 RECRUIT A WORKOUT BUDDY

Don't be tempted to give up your regular sessions. Organise workouts with a friend or colleague – ideally one who is a little above your own fitness level – to ensure you make it to every single session.

2 GET OUTSIDE

Exercising in your back garden or local park is a great way to beat gym boredom and boost your levels of mood-enhancing vitamin D.

3 UPDATE YOUR PLAYLIST

Listening to the same old songs over and over isn't a great way to motivate yourself. Ask your friends to share their favourite tracks with you and put together an upbeat workout compilation.

4 REVAMP YOUR KIT

Working out in old trackie bottoms is less than inspiring! You have to feel great to get the most out of your workout so invest in new threads for a boost.

5 REST UP

Take at least one rest day each week to allow your body to repair and to build strength. You'll be gagging to start again!

6 STAY INSPIRED

Stick a picture of an athlete who inspires you on your fridge to keep you motivated to stick to a healthy lifestyle.

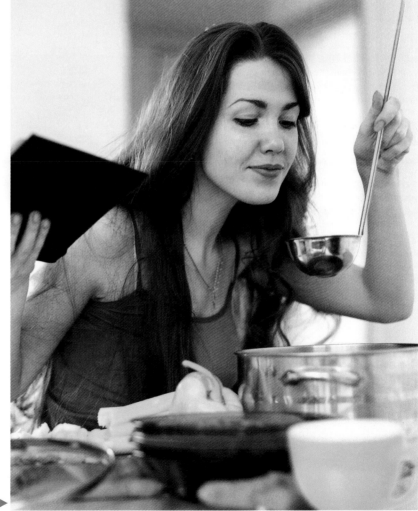

7 EAT UP

Make sure you have a carb-rich snack, such as a piece of toast and nut butter, before your workout and refuel with a protein shake.

8 GET KITTED OUT

A good pair of trainers is the one piece of kit you really can't scrimp on. Make sure you choose a shoe with cushioning and stability, and replace your trainers every six to 12 months.

9 DO SNEAKY WORKOUTS

Walk to work, take the stairs instead of the lift and cycle to the shops to blast away the calories without even noticing.

10 CHEAT IT

Stick to the 'cheat day' principle so you don't get into the habit of splurging on unhealthy food every day. A blowout once a week will give you something to look forward to and keeps your waistline in check.

11 KEEP A DIARY

Jot down your weekly goals and review them at the end of the week to help you stay focused. It's a great way to identify where you're struggling.

DON'T FORGET: EVERY MONTHLY ISSUE OF *WOMEN'S FITNESS* IS PACKED, NOT JUST WITH INSPIRING WORKOUTS, BUT HEALTHY RECIPES, LIFESTYLE ADVICE, BEAUTY TIPS AND MUCH MORE!

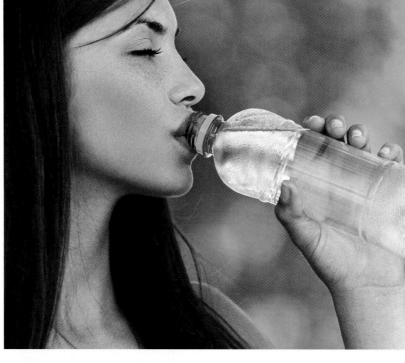

12 TREAT YOURSELF

Splash out on a manicure or massage when you feel like you've reached one of your key goals.

13 PLAN AHEAD

Cook a big batch of healthy meals and freeze them in single servings, to ensure you always have a nutritious option on hand when time is short.

14 STRETCH OUT

Make sure you do a dynamic stretching session before each workout to warm up your muscles. Go for moves that mimic the actions you'll be doing in your workout.

15 COOL DOWN

Stretch after each workout to reduce the risk of injury and muscle soreness. Use a foam roller to get deeper into your stretch.

16 BREATHE DEEP

Don't hold your breath when exercising! Good, deep breathing will help you stay focused and in control of every movement.

17 STAY HYDRATED

Your body loses fluid through sweat, so sip water at regular intervals to replenish the lost liquid. Aim for a minimum of two litres per day and one extra litre on workout days.

18 DON'T SKIP SESSIONS

Perform a good ratio of resistance and cardio training for a healthy balance that will keep your figure honed and toned.